Make the Pool Your Gym

2nd EDITION

T0017389

Make the Pool Your Gym

2nd EDITION

No-Impact Water Workouts for Getting Fit, Building Strength, and Rehabbing from Injury

Dr. Karl Knopf

ULYSSES PRESS

Published by:
Ulysses Press
PO Box 3440
Berkeley, CA 94703
www.ulyssespress.com

ISBN: 978-1-64604-507-5
Library of Congress Control Number: 2011934782

Printed in the United States by Kingery Printing Company
10 9 8 7 6 5 4 3 2 1

Acquisitions: Kierra Sondereker
Managing editor: Claire Chun
Editor: Renee Rutledge
Proofreader: Barbara Schultz
Front cover design: what!design @ whatweb.com
Photographs: © Alan Chun except page 15 webbed gloves © franctic00/
    shutterstock.com, jogger belt © Pashin Georgiy/shutterstock.com, water
    shoes/shutterstock.com; page 16 © Molotok289/shutterstock.com; page 22 ©
    marema/shutterstock.com
Models: Kitty Chiu, Chris Knopf, Karl Knopf, Sasha Wozniak
Production: Winnie Liu

Contents

PART 1: GETTING STARTED   **7**

Introduction: Water Workouts for All 9

Why Water Exercise? 10

Benefits of Water Fitness 12

The Evolution of Water Exercise 15

The Properties of Aqua Physics 17

Water Temperature 20

Before You Begin 21

PART 2: WORKOUTS   **27**

How to Use This Book 28

Sample Water Workouts 32

     General Fitness 33

     Advanced General Conditioning 35

     Sports Conditioning 37

Deep-Water Workout 39

     Arthritis 41

     Frozen Shoulder 43

     Low Back Pain 44

     Hip 46

     Knee 47

     Shin Splints 48

     Ankle/Feet 49

     Freeflow Routine 1 50

     Freeflow Routine 2 50

PART 3: THE EXERCISES   **51**

Warm-Up

     Water Walking 52

     Sideways Walking 53

     Skipping 54

Upper-Body Series

     Chest Press 55

     Fly 56

     Lateral Raise 57

     Frontal Raise 58

     Chest Tap 59

     Washboard 60

Lower-Body Series

     Forward Leg Raise 61

     Backward Leg Raise 62

     1-2-3 Leg Raise & Hold 63

     Side Leg Raise 64

     Leg Curl 65

     Leg Extension 66

     Heel Raise 67

     Toe Lift 68

Cardiovascular Conditioning 69

     Arm Add-Ons 69

     Leg Movements 77

     Jumping Sequence 84

Deep-Water Series

     Deep-Water Jogging 88

     Cross-Country Skiing 89

     Straight-Leg Kicks 90

     Soccer Kicks 91

     Deep-Water Sit-Ups 92

     Twist 93

     Rock Around the World 94

Stretches

     Hamstring Stretch 95

     Calf Stretch 95

     Ankle Circles 96

     Elbow Touches 97

     Double Wood Chop 98

     Shoulder Stretch 98

     Wrist Stretch 1 99

     Wrist Stretch 2 99

     Lower Back Stretch 100

Exercises Index 101

Acknowledgments 104

About the Author 104

PART 1

Getting Started

Introduction: Water Workouts for All

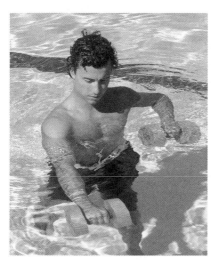

For years many fitness enthusiasts shied away from water fitness workouts because they believed that a water workout would not be challenging enough—wrong! A water workout, when designed correctly with the proper dose, provides the ideal exercise. Today we are seeing more highly fit men and women participating in water workouts. In *Make the Pool Your Gym*, I show you how to exercise in the pool and how to match your ability to the right exercises to obtain the ideal results. The ability to swim is not required, and you don't even need to get your hair wet. Water workouts provide a sensible and comprehensive way to exercise without subjecting the body to the same stress that's placed on it during land-based programs.

The beauty of water exercise is that it can accommodate the fitness needs of everyone. Many options exist to satisfy all levels and needs. Popular water workout options include:

Water aerobics: a fitness alternative to land-based exercise. Water aerobics feature vertical exercises like dancing, walking, running, jumping jacks, and kickboxing, as well as using resistance devices on the hands and ankles to foster muscular strength and endurance.

Deep water exercise: a nonimpact, high-intensity workout that helps prevent injuries from overuse and works as an effective method to recover from an injury.

Holistic workouts: performing exercise routines like yoga, Pilates , and tai chi moves in the water.

Sport-specific workouts: these include circuit training, shadow boxing, soccer kicks, cross-country skiing, or even tennis swings.

Adapted aquatics: water workouts designed to help individuals with disabilities or challenges.

Whether you're a serious athlete, a fitness enthusiast, a beginner, or someone with a chronic condition, water exercise can efficiently improve cardiovascular performance and strength in a very short amount of time. It's ideal for cross training, a total-body workout, and maintaining fitness in hot climates, and can also be used as an introductory mode of exercise.

Make the Pool Your Gym invites you to explore this safe and effective alternative way to get—and stay—fit. If you're tired of workouts that leave you feeling more battered than better, water workouts may be the solution.

Why Water Exercise?

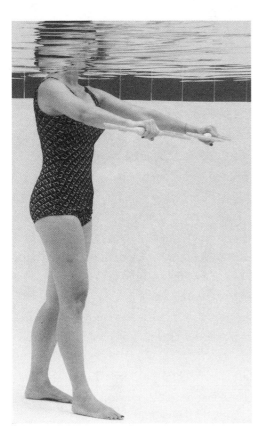

Numerous studies consistently support the idea that an improvement in fitness can contribute to an ever-widening set of health and economic benefits. Sedentary behaviors are associated with negative changes to the human body that can be reversed with modest exertion. This is where water exercise comes in. Physical activity/water exercise has been shown to improve health and functional fitness levels. Water exercise, in addition to physiological benefits, provides both social and psychological benefits. Engaging in a water workout can provide a safe and enjoyable mode of exercise.

Advantages of Water Fitness over Land Exercise

Water workouts offer numerous advantages over land workouts. Some high-level trainers use water as a method to engage in sports conditioning or as a way to employ plyometrics (training exercises that involve movements where muscles exert both speed and force in short intervals of time—like jumping—with the goal of increasing your muscle power.) Since water is far denser than air, water can apply up to 12 times greater resistance. The harder you push and pull during a water workout, the more productive it becomes. The resistance of water challenges everyone from beginners to highly conditioned athletes alike. Fortunately, water workouts have a built-in safety feature that land workouts lack. Since the amount of resistance in water depends on the speed of movement, you can't create more resistance than your body can tolerate.

Heart rates during water exercise are lower than during land-based training but you can still obtain the same physiological benefits with less heart-pounding exercise. Despite this, the common belief that water workouts burn less fat and fewer calories than other exercise is false. Aquatic aerobics can burn 400 to 700 calories an hour—about the same as land-based aerobics, but all without placing any strain on the joints while stimulating circulation. One recent study found that a one-hour water exercise session performed at a moderate pace expends the same amount of calories as walking for one hour at a pace of 3 miles per hour.

While swimming is an excellent vehicle for building muscle tone and endurance, it's limited to using the same set of muscles over and over again. Water exercise offers far more options and goes from horizontal to vertical, thus providing a comprehensive workout in multiple planes. This means participants can perform motions in any and all angles not available on standard exercise machines. The goal of any well-rounded workout is to provide a total-body workout that engages major muscle groups. Because water provides natural resistance to body movements, water exercises strengthen complementary muscle groups simultaneously. No land-based routine is as time efficient.

A Kinder, Gentler Way to Fitness

A decade ago, aqua exercise classes were few and far between and, when people heard the term "water exercise," they thought of residents at the retirement home doing simple moves. Today, water exercise is no longer just for seniors. While water is the perfect element for people with joint problems to exercise in because it diminishes the effects of gravity and allows movements that would be painful and difficult on land to be performed with greater ease, it also offers several more advantages over land, including greater buoyancy and better resistance, plus it's a whole lot more enjoyable.

Standing in neck-deep water, a person weighs about 10 percent of what he or she does on land. This effect, coupled with the cushioning property of water, places less pressure on the joints. This is especially beneficial to arthritis sufferers, athletes with joint or overuse injuries, and overweight people. Weekend warriors who are beat up from overtraining but won't take a day off for fear of deconditioning might consider cross training in water to maintain their fitness level. Some athletes can improve performance by taking time off to cross train in the pool. Non-impact deep-water running, for instance, has been proven to successfully hasten cardiovascular performance in athletes with overuse injuries.

Please note, however, that while water exercise is good for most people, there are some conditions under which water workouts should not be performed:
- Severe hypertension or hypotension
- Cardiac conditions
- Infectious skin disorders

It's always wise to consult your health-care professional for your specific recommendations.

Benefits of Water Fitness

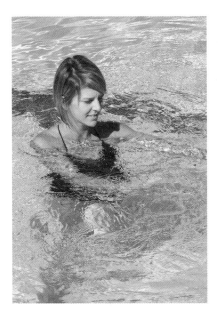

Recent research has shown that many of the health conditions seen today can be positively influenced by regular exercise and proper nutrition. This is where water fitness enters the scene. Not only can it be performed by most of the population, but also it provides social and psychological benefits as well as physiological ones.

Water fitness has a long list of benefits and a very short list of risks. The aquatic environment is a safe, effective, and inexpensive way to preserve health and improve functional fitness. Water fitness is the open door to health and wellness for people who have limited abilities and chronic conditions. In addition to its role in rehabilitation and physical therapy, water exercise can also provide a strenuous workout for elite athletes.

Many health issues can be remediated through water exercise, such as musculoskeletal problems, neurological problems, cardio-pulmonary conditions, and ambulatory conditions. The beauty of the aqua environment is individuals with mobility issues find that exercising in the pool allows for greater freedom of movement. Those with chronic pain also often find water exercise to be an effective way to improve fitness and (especially in warmer water) find temporary relief.

Water workouts provide a sensible and comprehensive way to exercise without subjecting your body to the stresses that are placed on it during land-based programs. Small amounts of physical activity can provide big benefits both physiologically and psychologically. Today, thanks to Americans with Disability Act, many public pools have access ramps or wheelchair lifts that allow everyone to enter the aqua fitness environment.

Athletes and hard-core fitness enthusiasts will find that water exercise allows them to get a total body workout in half the time because they are using both agonist and antagonist muscles. A total body workout is also achievable if they use the aqua physics principles (see page 17 for more on aqua physics) to their advantage. Water exercise provides an excellent method to cross train when it is too hot to train outdoors, and even swimmers enjoy having the option to engage in water fitness as a break from the boredom of swimming laps.

Physiological Benefits
- Improved muscular strength and endurance
- Increased functional flexibility
- Expanded cardiovascular fitness
- Decreased pain
- Decreased impact on joints
- Decreased risk of injury
- Improved sleep patterns
- Hastened recovery time from injuries
- Better posture and body mechanics
- Reduced risk for chronic diseases

Social and Psychological Benefits
- Improved self-efficacy and self-esteem
- Reduced pain
- Increased social interaction and new friendships
- Opportunity to develop social support
- Reduced tension and stress
- Improved sleep
- Decreased fatigue

While water exercise is good for most people, there are some conditions under which water workouts should not be performed:
- Severe hypertension or hypotension
- Cardiac conditions
- Infectious skin disorders

It's always wise to consult your health-care professional for your specific recommendations. Water exercise is NOT a replacement for physical therapy or medical treatment.

Research Supporting Water Fitness Benefits

Numerous studies support the advantages of water exercise. Water fitness can have a positive influence on body composition and encourage weight loss. Water workouts burn calories just like any other form of exercise when done at comparable intensity levels. Since caloric expenditure is based on both intensity and duration, aquatic aerobics can burn about the same number of calories as land-based aerobics, all without placing any strain on the joints and still stimulating circulation.

A study in 2019 found that aquatic exercise helped relieve chronic back pain more effectively than land-based programs. Another study found that water exercise has been proven to be helpful for pregnant women experiencing back pain.

Heart rates during water exercise are lower than during land-based training, but you can still obtain the same physiological benefits with less heart-pounding exercise.

An interesting study found that water aerobics improved cognitive function in older adults. The premise is, what is good for the heart is good for the brain.

An encouraging study published in *The Harvard Health Letter* reported that those 85 years and older who regularly practiced a healthy lifestyle behavior and were involved in a water exercise program live longer and have fewer years of dementia.

Small amounts of physical activity can provide big benefits. Even low levels of physical activity at less than 150 minutes per week can reduce depression. (If you can engage in water exercise with a friend, the social benefits are even better.)

Aerobic fitness level is a greater predictor of longevity than age alone.

Or said another way, the longer you go without regular exercise, the more likely you are to have dementia, diabetes, and/or high blood pressure.

Exercising in a warm pool reduces pain and stiffness, and improves the function of people with hip and knee arthritis. Water workouts increase muscular strength in those with chronic arthritis.

Bottom line: If it's physical it's therapy—move it or lose it!

The Evolution of Water Exercise

Water therapy/fitness has been around since 200 BC. Much of the current field of aquatic rehabilitation has its roots in the European and early American spa world. Social bathing was also an important part of ancient Greek and Roman culture. Since earliest recorded history, water has been believed to promote healing and has been widely used in the management of medical ailments.

Natural springs and water therapies became a central focus of many health spas and healers, who noted the positive effects of water on various medical conditions. It's through observation and centuries of trial and error that today's scientific methodology of aquatic treatments have evolved.

No Special Equipment Needed

No special equipment is needed to get a tremendous water workout. Back in the early days of water exercise, the only method to change resistance was simply to alter the angle of your hands or modify the speed of your movement. Those methods are still useful and can provide an effective water workout.

In the 1980s, empty milk jugs were used in water exercise to add to the experience, until the health departments said that they were unsanitary. Then along came some ingenious entrepreneurs who invented resistance-training devices such as plastic hand paddles, webbed gloves, and ankle paddles.

As deep-water exercises like aqua jogging became popular, even more helpful equipment was invented, including noodles and aqua jogger belts for those who found treading water too difficult.

As more and more people engaged in vertical aqua aerobics, they found that the pool bottoms were rough on their feet. At first, people would simply wear their regular running shoes while working out in the pool, but this practice was unsanitary (not to mention it took days for the shoes to dry out). Fortunately, creative entrepreneurs designed aqua jogging shoes that would provide foot support and protection during water workouts, while also drying quickly.

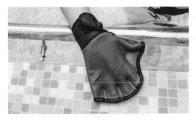
Webbed gloves for aqua aerobics

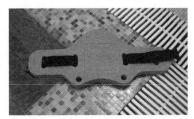
Jogger belt for aqua jogging

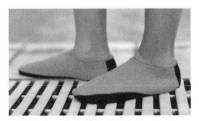
Water shoes for aqua aerobics

Make Your Pool a Gym

In the early days of water fitness, finding space to perform water exercise was limited, as swimmers did not want to share their pool with water fitness folks. Fortunately, today you don't need to belong to a class or swim club to participate in the water fitness experience. For the price of a stand-alone pool, you can have your own home water fitness gym.

Any pool that is 4 to 5 feet deep and approximately 6x6 feet is all that is needed. Stand-alone pools can be installed above or below ground. And if you are worried about the cost of heating the pool, wearing a wet suit can make any pool useable. Some people who live in cooler climates even enclose the pool or have it installed in the garage.

For a list of water exercise equipment vendors, check out https://aeawave.org/Shop/eSource-Guide.

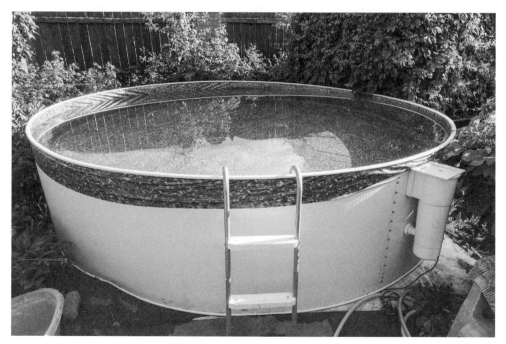

Stand-alone pool for aqua aerobics

The Properties of Aqua Physics

Water workouts offer numerous advantages over land workouts. Some high-level athletes use water as a method to engage in cross training to break up the wear and tear of a land-based routine. Since water is far denser than air, water can apply up to 12 times greater resistance. The harder you push and pull during a water workout, the more productive it becomes. Using the water resistance properly can benefit and challenge both untrained and highly conditioned athletes. The secret to obtaining the benefits of a water workout is to know how and when to employ aqua physics to elicit the correct outcome. You don't need to be an expert in hydrodynamics, but understanding the basic properties of water can influence the design of your water exercise session.

SAFETY FIRST

Fortunately, water workouts have a built-in safety feature that land workouts lack. Too often on weight machines in the gym, a simple misstep or adding too much weight to the machine can cause an injury. Since the amount of resistance in water depends entirely on your speed of movement, you can't create more resistance than your body can tolerate.

Land vs. Water

Too many land exercisers think that water exercise is just land exercises done in the pool. However, the forces applied in the water are very different from those on land. As an example, clap your hands quickly together and spread them apart on land, then do that same movement in the water. You'll see how, when performed in the water, resistance is applied throughout the full range of motion in both directions. Now, straighten your hand and repeat the same movement, slicing through the water. Then do this again with a cupped hand. Repeat each movement both fast and slow. Now you have an understanding of aqua-dynamics, that is, that water can be used to both assist movements as well as act as a resistance force.

Overview of the Principles of Water Fitness

There are a number of principles, such as buoyancy, drag, turbulence, and water temperature, that will impact your water workout. The following is a brief overview of the major influencers seen in water fitness.

Take a Load Off: Buoyancy

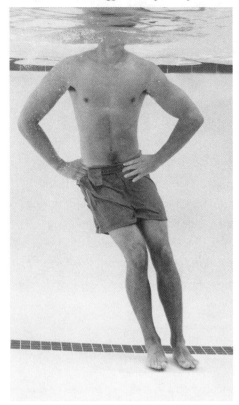

When performing exercise on land, gravity is the primary force you must overcome. Buoyancy gives water exercise its "soft" capacity, which reduces compression and weight bearing on joints. This is why water exercise can be a great option for those who are obese or have orthopedic conditions. The deeper you stand in the water, the more buoyancy plays a role in lifting you off the floor of the pool. For instance, if you stand in neck-deep water, you'll weigh only 10 percent of your body weight; if you stand in waist-deep water, you'll weigh 50 percent of your body weight. Thus, the deeper you go, the less you weigh. This effect, coupled with the cushioning property of water, places less stress on the joints. This is especially beneficial to arthritis sufferers, athletes with joint or overuse injuries, and overweight people. Weekend warriors who are beat up from overtraining can consider cross training in water to maintain their fitness level while they recover without deconditioning. Some athletes can improve performance by taking time off to cross train in the pool. Non-impact deep-water running, for instance, has been proven to successfully prevent cardiovascular deconditioning in athletes with overuse injuries.

Drag

When in the water, drag is the resistance you encounter as you move through it. Drag is the primary force that governs your pace in the water. The faster you move in the water, the more drag you create. For the aquatic exerciser, drag and turbulence are beneficial tools for increasing resistance and building strength.

The larger the surface area or the faster the motion, the more drag gets generated, causing more resistance and challenges to the exerciser. An example is running as fast as you can while holding a kickboard perpendicular to the bottom of the pool. If you are a swimmer, you definitely understand the concept of drag; that is why a streamlined bathing suit is much easier to swim in than a baggy pair of pants.

Turbulence

The more abruptly you move through water, the more turbulence you'll create. A person who is physically limited may want to limit turbulence as much as possible to limit any additional resistance. An elite runner, on the other hand, may want to create as much turbulence as possible to increase resistance, which is not possible on land.

Viscosity

Viscosity of the water provides a natural resistive environment for exercise. When the body is submerged during aquatic exercise, it is affected by resistance in all directions of movement. Exploiting this beneficial property of water has an extreme impact on physical strength gains, especially when the force is against the directional motion.

Velocity

Velocity of the movement parallels the increase in resistance, which requires a higher level of work to complete the exercise. This results in more muscular effort to overcome the resistance.

Motion

Motion occurs when there's a change of location in space, and it can be linear or rotational. With water exercise, you can apply resistance in any direction that's physically possible.

Acceleration

Acceleration (the rate of change of velocity/speed) is one component of motion. It'll require more effort/power for you to apply a new sudden burst of movement than just continuing a movement at the same pace. This approach can be applied as a conditioning tool (for example, quickly running forward 5 feet, stopping, and reversing directions can be a challenging workout). Another advantage of water fitness is that it provides resistance in 3D, which makes it ideal for balance training and functional fitness training.

Cooling Effects

Water dissipates heat more effectively than on land. The chances of overheating in the pool are less, as water continuously cools the body. The ideal temperature for most water exercise sessions is 82°F. However, for those who become easily chilled in a pool, it may be a good idea to wear a wet suit.

Water Temperature

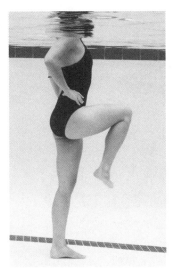

Water transfers heat or cold more quickly than air, which means a water temperature of 75°F will seem much colder than an air temperature of 75°F. Most experts agree that skin temperature is approximately 93°F and anything less than that is going to feel cooler to your skin.

Everyone has a preference when it comes to water temperature. A person with arthritis or joint pain will prefer warm water, a client with multiple sclerosis might prefer cooler water, while a person who wants a vigorous workout will tolerate a cooler water temperature.

Understanding the effects of water temperatures will increase your attendance rate and enjoyment. Most multipurpose pools are kept at 82°F. Keep in mind that swimmers generally like the pool cooler and, with the cost of energy getting higher it is not likely the pool temperature will ideally meet your wishes. If the pool temperature is not ideal, you may opt to wear a lightweight wet suit. Entry into the pool will almost always feel cool, so a shower beforehand or a light wet suit can make the transition easier.

The most comfortable temperature range for water aerobics is 80 to 84°F. If the pool is cooler than this, you'll need to do a thermal warmup for a longer time or wear a wet suit.

Pool temperatures warmer than 86 to 88°F can be hazardous for vigorous workouts.

Each type of workout has an ideal water temperature:
- Arthritis/therapy classes: 83–88°F
- Competitive athletic classes: 78–82°F
- Stretch and relax classes: 83–86°F

Resistance

Water provides continual resistance to every move you make. Water is 12 to 14 times more resistant than air. Water's resistance allows exercises to be easily and gradually adjusted based on speed, levers, and surface area. Just add a variable resistance-training device (VRTD) or simply open your hand to increase resistance. However, an open hand slicing through the water creates less intense movement than either a fist or an open hand that impacts the water with the palm.

Resistance exerted on the surface straight on is called "frontal tension." Because of frontal tension, walking forward is harder than walking sideways; it is also why you can more easily slice your hand through the water than slap it.

Before You Begin

As stated earlier, applying the principles of aqua physics can make a workout suitable for all levels of individuals. Water fitness can provide you with a total body workout. It can improve cardiorespiratory fitness, posture, and functional mobility, as well as tone muscles all at the same time. The beauty of a well-designed water exercise program is that it can work both agonist and antagonist muscle groups with just one simple exercise and engage muscles in directions and manners not possible with cables, dumbbells, or machines. This means you can work out your whole body in half the time—perfect for people with busy schedules. Some may joke it is a "no sweat workout."

Below is a chart that shows agonist and antagonist muscles groups.

OPPOSING MUSCLE GROUPS

Agonist	Antagonist
Abdominals	Erector spinae
Biceps brachii	Triceps brachii
Anterior deltoid	Posterior deltoid
Gastrocnemius	Tibialis anterior
Hamstring	Quadriceps
Pectoralis	Rhomboids & Mid-trapezius

Another advantage of water exercise is that it is isokinetic, which means that the resistance stays consistent through the full range of motion. This is not possible on conventional weight-training machines.

SAFETY FIRST

Before you start a water-fitness program, it's critical that you're water safe. Even though you don't need to be a swimmer, you need to be able to keep yourself above water and be able to swim/paddle to a safe area if you lose your footing. You also need to be able to enter and exit the pool safely. Once in the pool, most people feel so good they often overdo it. Start out very slowly and progress from a safe foundation. Always consult your physician before starting any exercise program.

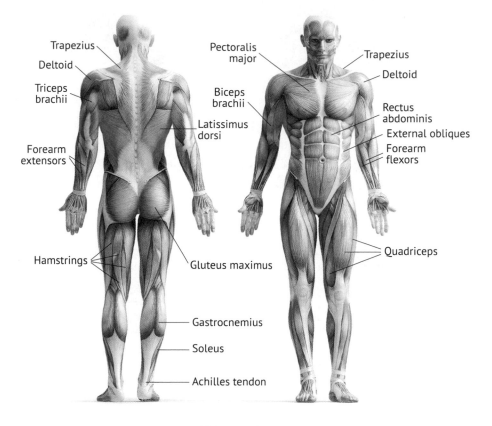

Major muscles

Be Heart Smart

Water exercise heart rates don't need to be as high as land-based exercise heart rates, so keep that in mind while you work out. The "talk test" is the best approach to follow when doing water exercise—if you can't talk while exercising, you're working too hard, but if you can debate a hot topic, you're not working hard enough. Remember: train, don't strain! As always, consult your health professional for any specific guidelines for your health condition. A prudent guideline is to monitor blood sugar levels pre/post exercise.

STAY UNDERWATER!

When performing water workouts, try to keep the majority of movements in the water. Having your arms out of the water will change your heart rate and influence your body mechanics. (When your arms are out of the water, your heart rate becomes artificially higher and doesn't provide a true representation of your exercise intensity.) More importantly, when your arms are out of the water, you're not applying any of the properties of water to your upper body. Bottom line: arm exercises out of the water should be limited.

Safety

The exercises contained in this book have been shown over time to be a safe and prudent method of exercise. However, keep in mind that chronic use of any movement can exacerbate an orthopedic condition. If an exercise is done too intensely or without following proper biomechanics, an injury can result.

While water exercise is generally safe for everyone, a few conditions (infectious skin disorders, severe high/low blood pressure, some heart issues, uncontrolled seizures) may be unsafe for an aquatic fitness environment. It's always wise when in doubt to consult a physician or physical therapist before performing water workouts. None of the programs included in this book are intended to replace physical therapy.

Safety Tips for an Enjoyable and Satisfying Water Workout

Let's review certain protocols that should be taken to have a great, safe workout.

1. Always make sure your body is ready for movement with an adequate warmup.
2. Find the correct depth of the water where you can maintain proper posture.
3. If exercising outdoors, stay alert to air quality and pollution, and make sure you protect your skin.
4. Remember to breathe normally during exercise—don't hold your breath! Many people unknowingly do this while performing the strength portion of a water exercise class. Counting, talking, or singing along with the movement encourages breathing.
5. Some water aerobics classes use music in their program. Consider standing away from the speakers to preserve your hearing and to actually hear the instructor's commands.
6. When you're done with the high-intensity portion of your workout, continue with low-intensity exercise (such as water walking) to encourage the proper return of blood to your heart and normal breathing. This will prevent any "pooling" effect that may occur in the lower extremities.
7. Never leave the water exercise session while having an exercise-induced raised heart rate or jump into a hot shower, sauna, or hot tub while still having an elevated heart rate.
8. Train, don't strain. It does not have to hurt to be fit.
9. Remember the two-hour rule: evaluate how you feel two hours post exercise. If you feel uncomfortable or worse post exercise, back off exercising for a bit and possibly consult your health professional if serious concerns present themselves.
10. Make your program functional to meet your goals, but keep "fun" in functional. We tend to repeat those activities that are enjoyable. Regular fitness needs to be a lifetime commitment. With time, adapt your water fitness program to meet your current goals, mood, etc.
11. Listen to your body and never overdo it.
12. Remember to use the FIT concept to improve fitness and function:
    - **F** = Frequency; regular exercise is important to see results.
    - **I** = Intensity; this needs to be just right, too much increases the chance of injury and not enough may not provide results.
    - **T** = Time; the duration needs to be long enough to obtain the desired objective.

Many professional and world-class athletes use water to maintain their fitness when injured. Some factors to keep in mind when using water to rehabilitate a sports injury:

- Follow the advice of a physician and/or therapist.
- Exercise unaffected areas until you're approved for exercising injured areas.
- Cross train—exercise both agonist and antagonist muscle groups.
- Develop your workout to exercise muscles that replicate the specific sport requirements and movements.
- If a movement is painful, slow down the movement and decrease the range of motion.
- Make increases in resistance and speed slowly.
- Use visualization, variations, and fun to keep workouts enjoyable and challenging.

Exercises to Be Careful With

Even if you think you're in great physical shape, you should still pay attention to your body when performing water workouts. All it takes is one wrong movement to give yourself an injury or to exacerbate a chronic condition. Possible high-risk areas include the shoulders, low back, hips, and knees.

Arms/Shoulders

- Straighten arms smoothly—avoid hyperextending or hyperflexing the elbow joint (this means no snapping the arms to an extreme straight position) and avoid jerky motions.
- Keep your hands where you can see them. Any time your hands are out of sight, you're at potential risk of causing trauma to the shoulder joint.
- Avoid adding resistance equipment before you're ready. For best results, do exercises with arms in the water.

Low Back

- Regardless of the movement you perform, you should always maintain good neutral spine posture.
- Perform straight-leg swings slowly and with control to prevent your spine from twisting; keep your core engaged.
- When doing flutter kicks while holding onto a kickboard or the edge of the pool, keep your back, neck, and shoulders protected. Some people find using a snorkel helpful in preventing the low back from arching excessively.

Hips

- Perform straight-leg extensions slowly and smoothly, and only raise the leg to hip height.
- Bringing your knees higher than hip height or 90° may cause issues if you have hip problems or osteoporosis.
- Be careful with crossing leg motions or taking legs too far to the side.

Knees

- Avoiding using resistance devices on your legs if you have knee issues.
- Keep your knee centered over your ankle and bent no more than 90° when lunging to the front. Use extreme caution when doing lateral side steps.
- Be careful when twisting, pivoting, or performing cutting motions, as these can cause additional stress to the knee joint.
- Avoid hyper-flexing or hyperextending the leg.

Exercise Basics

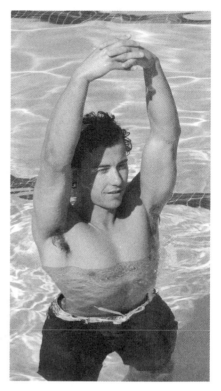

As stated earlier, you don't need any special equipment to reap the benefits of water exercise. Both an open hand and a closed fist can generate adequate resistance to give you a good workout. The secrets to effective water exercise are the three S's: speed (the faster you move, the more resistance you generate), size/surface area (the larger the surface area of the object, the more resistance), and shape of the object.

If you are new to exercise, the following are some basic terms you may hear through this book and as you advance through your exercise journey.

Physical activity: can include exercise but it also relates to purposeful and functional activities of daily living, such as getting around, gardening, grocery shopping, or gaining full employment. Exercise is a subset of physical activity.

Hypokinetic disease: conditions that can arise through too little exercise or movement. Being sedentary is now considered as big a risk factor to your health as smoking. Poor diet and lack of exercise lead to metabolic syndrome conditions such as diabetes and heart disease.

Exercise: a term that implies a regular, repetitive approach to physical activity.

Repetitions: the number of times you perform an exercise to complete a set.

Set: a grouping of repetitions.

Interval training: going hard for a specific amount of time and then taking a specific rest period.

HIT: high-intensity interval training.

Flexibility: the ability to move the joint through its normal range of motion. Flexibility is very important and there are different types of stretching methods to improve flexibility. Stretching is important for the maintenance of mobility and overall function of the body.

It has been said: Stretch what is tight and strengthen what is lax. Flexibility is often neglected in a total body exercise session, so make sure not to skip this important step.

Dynamic stretching: gently moving the body through a pain-free, full range of motion in a slow controlled manner. The key aspect of this type of stretching is to stay within the safe range of motion. Dynamic stretching is usually a good way to prepare the joint and body for movement.

Ballistic stretching: generally a bouncing stretch that involves using momentum to force the body past its safe range of motion, which is often not recommended for most people, especially as a warmup.

Static stretching: moving the joint to the end range of motion and holding it there for 30 seconds to a minute to a mild level of discomfort. This is best done after thermal warmup or at the end of your exercise session.

Strength training: exercise that involves using land-resistance training devices such as handheld weights, exercise machines, a person's body weight, or resistance training devices in the pool. Too often, we lose muscular strength with age if not engaged in a sensible progressive resistance exercise program.

PRE (Progressive resistance training): as a muscle gets stronger, you apply more resistance in your exercise.

Cardiovascular training, **cardio respiratory training**, or **aerobics:** terms that are used almost interchangeably. To obtain cardiovascular fitness, a person needs to train at a target heart rate for a specific amount of time.

Thermal warm-up: done to increase your core temperature and prepare your muscles for motion. After the body is warm, then flexibility exercises can be employed.

Strength: generally attained by doing a heavier/harder amount of resistance with fewer repetitions (6 to 10).

Muscular endurance: generally attained by doing a higher number of repetitions (10 to 20).

PART 2
Workouts

How to Use This Book

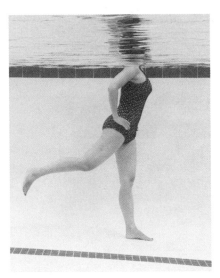

The goal of *Make the Pool Your Gym* is to help you regain or maintain range of motion, cardiovascular fitness, and strength without overdoing it. To avoid injury, this book offers you methods for a total body workout that address all aspects of fitness. Don't let anybody "should" on you! Train at an intensity that feels best for you! Remember the two-hour rule: If you feel worse two hours post-exercise, evaluate what you did and delete an exercise or decrease the intensity or the time of your workout.

This next section of *Make the Pool Your Gym* presents workouts (starting on page 32) for a number of training goals and physical conditions. Pick the one that best suits your needs, or use the samples as springboards for creating your own routine. The following sample workouts are designed so that you start with a warm-up and progress to more advanced exercises. All exercise descriptions are provided in Part 3. If you prefer creating your own workout, you can do that too. Just add water and have fun with fitness! No two people are exactly the same, so feel free to adapt and individualize the programs to meet your specific desires.

Designing a Water-Fitness Workout

The beauty of a water-fitness program is that there really are no rules. No one can see what's going on below the surface so, as long as you feel fine, go for it. Your body and the water will tell you what's best for you. Too often water-fitness instructors make up complicated routines solely for the purpose of keeping themselves from getting bored. Your heart, lungs, and muscles don't care if the routine is choreographed or basic. The perfect workout is the one you enjoy while you're doing it, and makes you feel good afterward.

Some people enjoy simply turning on music and moving in a free-form manner. To keep from getting bored, change the exercise after every song, or every 30 seconds or every minute. You can also take your step aerobics program or your dance aerobics program and perform it in the pool. Some individuals enjoy doing calisthenic routines in the pool, such as jogging in place and doing jumping jacks, cross-country skiing or explosive jumps.

Feel free to mix and match your favorite leg exercises with your favorite arm movements; and switch the combinations around depending on how your body feels or responds to the exercises. Another fun option is keeping the leg motions constant for five minutes and change the arms motion every one minute. After that, include new leg motions and start all over. Most people have chosen water exercise for a reason, perhaps because their joints hurt, or they have overtrained on land, or just for a change of venue. When it comes to water fitness, enjoy the process—be creative and playful. Again, as long as you're enjoying yourself and avoiding injury, *Make the Pool your Gym* has no rules.

While the above may sound fine for some, I know many people want guidelines. Here are some suggestions for designing a fun and fabulous fitness workout. A sample routine might look something like this:

- Thermal warm-up session: 5–10 minutes.
- Aerobic activity: 20–30 minutes at a comfortable intensity.
- Strength training/conditioning: 10–15 minutes.
- Post-workout cool down, stretching: 5–10 minutes; focus on working the major muscles in the body.
- Relaxation: if desired, as long as you stay comfortable.

The order of aerobics and strength training portions can be switched, and the duration of each activity can be lengthened as desired.

Start with a Thermal Warm-Up

Begin with a thermal warm-up to increase your core temperature and prepare your muscles for motion. Usually, this takes 5–10 minutes and includes water walking in all directions with various arms motions. I also call this portion "inventory check-in time." While you walk, check which parts of your body are clicking and which parts are clunking. After the inventory check, you should know which parts of your body need TLC that day. Many people like to spend a few minutes after the thermal warm-up to do some extra gentle moves/stretches to ready the body for movement. If you feel fine, just progress to the next section of your routine, but make sure you stretch at the end of your routine to foster your flexibility, whether you do so in the pool or the hot tub, or on land.

Train with Your Goal in Mind

A workout session with specific goals and objectives has a better chance of achieving the specific results.

To achieve your desired results and stay motivated, determine and write down your long-term fitness goals, then write down objectives and how you plan to achieve those goals.

Example:

Goal: I want to lose 20 pounds in one year.

Objective: I plan to lose two pounds per month.

Pre-test: What is your current weight? Write it down.

Post-test: Measure your weight weekly to see how you are progressing. If you obtain your objectives and goals, reward yourself. If not, evaluate what needs to change.

If your focus is increased range of motion in specific joints, perform the gentle motions that address your needs.

If your focus is cardiovascular fitness and weight management, the aerobic exercise session should be 30–40 minutes of cardiovascular movements. This can be a combination of shallow- and deep-water exercises, or just one type. After your cardio workout, spend 1–5 minutes allowing your heart to return to your pre-exercise heart rate. Remember: Aquatic heart rates are about 10–15 beats per minute less than your terrestrial target heart rate. If the air quality is poor or pool temperature is too warm, skip this portion and do some gentle stretches or balance work instead; otherwise, progress directly to resistance work.

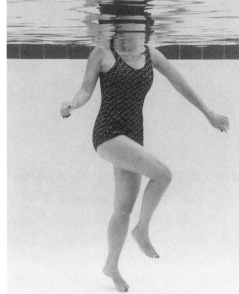

If your goal is to tone and strengthen your body, find a resistance that challenges your muscles so that by 30 seconds (10–20 repetitions), your muscles feel like they've been exercised. Eventually work up to doing three sets of 30 seconds at a moderate speed then go faster and faster. Keep in mind the three S's (see 25) as a way to increase resistance. You should be able to recover in 30–60 seconds or sooner before you do the next set. Some people prefer to do a complete series of all the exercises and then repeat the whole sequence again, or target one area before moving on to the next (e.g., three sets of chest, then three sets of shoulders, etc.). You can even design a circuit in which you move across the pool doing one exercise for 30 seconds, then move across to the other side doing another exercise and so on. Note that if you're doing a land-based weight-training program, there's no need to do resistance training in an aquatic environment.

Perform a Cooldown After Each Session

Stretching and cooling down after your water workout is as important to your exercise routine as warming up before your workout. A sudden cessation of aerobic activity may cause blood to pool in your lower extremities, which deprives the brain and heart of oxygenated blood and can cause light-headedness or nausea. Thus, it's critical to allow your breathing and heart rate to return pre-exercise levels. To perform your cooldown, walk slowly back and forth in the pool or just swim at a very relaxed pace for about five minutes or until your heart rate returns to the pre-exercise level.

Safety Tip: Never jump into the hot tub, bath, or shower until you have regained your pre-exercise heart rate and breathing frequency. If exercising alone, always have a phone nearby in case of an emergency. And always use caution while walking around slippery pool decks!

Finish with Stretching

Concentrate on the large muscles, such as hamstrings, calves, shoulders, and lower back. Stay mindful that when stretching in the pool you may get chilled, so holding the stretch for as long as it's needed may not be possible. Therefore, you may opt for doing your stretching program on land after your water workout.

Some people really enjoy doing a mindful relaxation/meditation session at the end of their exercise routine. A relaxing stretch at the end of your water workout can have a profound healing effect in terms of restoring the body, mind, and spirit. Combining the benefits of stretching, meditation, and relaxation is a wonderful way to complete a total body workout. Deep breathing as you relax is designed to get you to connect mind and body. You can try this by floating in the pool with a flotation device under your arms and focusing on breathing and decompressing your spine.

Here are some stretching tips:

- Perform stretches while breathing slowly and rhythmically in through your nose and out through your mouth.
- To avoid straining ligaments, keep all joints slightly bent/flexed while moving in a controlled manner and in proper alignment. Protect your spine at all times (i.e., keep your knees relaxed and your pelvis tilted).
- Stretch to the point of mild tension and try to hold for 10–60 seconds. Don't bounce.
- Repeat all stretches 1–3 times (depending on your abilities). Each time you stretch, try to go a bit further or hold a little longer, if possible. It might be wise to pay particular attention to problem areas.
- If any stretch hurts, stop! Listen to your body and trust your ability to distinguish between pain and a good stretch.

The stretching series, designed to improve flexibility and prevent injury, is best done at the end of a workout, although some people like performing a few gentle stretches after a warm-up. The choice is yours—listen to your body.

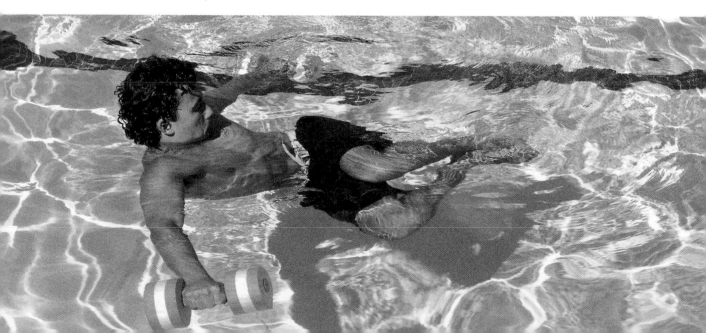

Sample Water Workouts

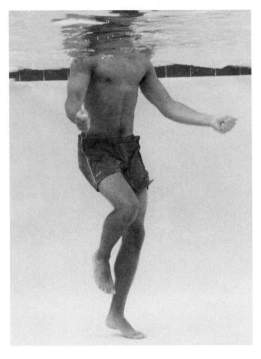

Here are some workouts to get you started. Consider them suggestions. If any move doesn't feel good, try a different angle or a different exercise—your body will tell you what's right for you if you listen. The first thing you may notice when you go through one of these workouts is the omission of repetitions (reps) and sets. Unfortunately, most of us are still dialed into the outdated mind-set of "How many do you want me to do, Coach?"

When deciding how many reps or sets of these exercises to do, the key is to forget about the number of reps you need to do and, instead, focus on maintaining proper posture and engaging the targeted muscles. You'll get better results by tuning in to your body and performing the movements with correct biomechanical form.

If that concept is too far out for you, start with 3–5 reps for active movements or 10 seconds for static positions. As the movement becomes easy, add more reps or think of other methods to challenge yourself. Aim to increase the number of reps to 30 or hold static poses for 30–60 seconds. Remember, more is not necessarily better. Also, when performing the movements, focus on breathing and being centered.

(For more information on designing your own personalized routine, please turn to page 28.) Now turn on some music and enjoy the freedom a total-body water workout affords you!

General Fitness

This routine is designed for an entry-level person looking for a total-body workout. It allows you to move in a pain-free manner. Don't force a move; if it doesn't feel good, don't do it. After class you shouldn't feel any worse than when you started. If you do, back off a bit next time but don't quit.

WARM-UP

EXERCISE	PAGE	DURATION
Water Walking	52	1 minute
Sideways Walking	53	1 minute
Skipping	54	1 minute

CARDIOVASCULAR CONDITIONING

EXERCISE	PAGE	DURATION
High Steps with Breaststroke Arms	77 / 69	3–5 minutes
High Steps with Fly Arms	77 / 71	3–5 minutes
High Steps with Punching	77 / 72	3–5 minutes
Jumping Jacks with Jumping Jack Arms: Side	78 / 76	3–5 minutes
Jumping Jacks with Punching	78 / 72	3–5 minutes
Cross-Country Skiing with Cross-Country Arms	79 / 73	3–5 minutes

UPPER-BODY CONDITIONING

EXERCISE	PAGE	DURATION
Chest Press	55	30 seconds
Lateral Raise	57	30 seconds
Chest Tap	59	30 seconds

LOWER-BODY CONDITIONING

EXERCISE	PAGE	DURATION
Forward Leg Raise	61	30 seconds
Side Leg Raise	64	30 seconds
Heel Raise	67	30 seconds

STRETCHING

EXERCISE	PAGE	DURATION
Hamstring Stretch	95	30 seconds
Calf Stretch	95	30 seconds
Elbow Touches	97	30 seconds

Advanced General Conditioning

You can try this routine if you're relatively fit, injury-free and/or proficient in water exercise.

WARM-UP

EXERCISE	PAGE	DURATION
Water Walking	52	1 minute
Sideways Walking	53	1 minute
Skipping	54	1 minute

CARDIOVASCULAR CONDITIONING

EXERCISE	PAGE	DURATION
Cross-Country Skiing with Jumping Jack Arms: Side	79 / 76	1–5 minutes
Cross-Country Skiing with Piston Arms	79 / 71	1–5 minutes
Straight-Leg Kicks with Breaststroke Arms	80 / 69	1–5 minutes
Straight-Leg Kicks with Paddlewheels	80 / 74	1–5 minutes
Soccer Kicks with Hug Arms	81 / 70	1–5 minutes
Soccer Kicks with Fly Arms	81 / 71	1–5 minutes
Rock Around the World (deep-water)	94	1–5 minutes
6 o'clock to 12 o'clock Jumps	85	1–5 minutes
9 o'clock to 3 o'clock Jumps	86	1–5 minutes
High Steps with Paddlewheels	77 / 74	1–5 minutes

UPPER-BODY CONDITIONING

EXERCISE	PAGE	DURATION
Frontal Raise	58	1 minute
Washboard	60	1 minute
Punching	72	1 minute
Chest Tap	59	1 minute

LOWER-BODY CONDITIONING

EXERCISE	PAGE	DURATION
Leg Curl	65	1 minute
Forward Leg Raise	61	1 minute
Backward Leg Raise	62	1 minute
Side Leg Raise	64	1 minute
Leg Extension	66	1 minute
Rocking Horse	83	1 minute

STRETCHING

EXERCISE	PAGE	DURATION
Hamstring Stretch	95	30 seconds
Calf Stretch	95	30 seconds
Elbow Touches	97	30 seconds

Sports Conditioning

This routine is designed for those who like to challenge themselves, are cross training, or are recovering from a sports injury.

WARM-UP

EXERCISE	PAGE	DURATION
Water Walking	52	1 minute
Sideways Walking	53	1 minute
Skipping	54	1 minute
Jump Rope	87	1 minute

CARDIOVASCULAR CONDITIONING *do three sets*

EXERCISE	PAGE	DURATION
High Steps with Chest Tap Arms	77 / 75	15–30 seconds
High Steps with Jumping Jack Arms: Frontal	77 / 76	15–30 seconds
High Steps with Washboard Arms	77 / 70	15–30 seconds
High Steps with Arm Circles each direction	77 / 73	15–30 seconds
Underwater Rockets	84	15–30 seconds
Cross-Country Skiing with Fly Arms	79 / 71	15–30 seconds
Cross-Country Skiing with Cross-Country Arms	79 / 73	15–30 seconds
Soccer Kicks with Jumping Jack Arms: Side	81 / 76	15–30 seconds

UPPER-BODY CONDITIONING *do three sets, max intensity*

EXERCISE	PAGE	DURATION
Punching	72	1 minute
Fly	56	1 minute
Chest Tap	59	1 minute
Lateral Raise	57	1 minute
Washboard	60	1 minute
Frontal Raise	58	1 minute

LOWER-BODY CONDITIONING *do three sets, max intensity*

EXERCISE	PAGE	DURATION
Straight-Leg Kicks	80	1 minute
Butt Kickers	82	1 minute
Soccer Kicks	81	1 minute
Heel Raise	67	1 minute
Toe Lift	68	1 minute
Side Leg Raise	64	1 minute

COOLDOWN AND STRETCHING

EXERCISE	PAGE	DURATION
Water Walking	52	5–10 min
Sideways Walking	53	5–10 min
Skipping	54	5–10 min
Hamstring Stretch	95	hold 30 seconds
Calf Stretch	95	hold 30 seconds
Elbow Touches	97	hold 30 seconds

Deep-Water Workout

This routine can be ideal for people with joint considerations or it can be very challenging for the elite athlete. It's an excellent way to cross train between difficult land-based activities like basketball, running, and tennis. The critical elements are intensity and duration.

This method allows you to keep your aerobic fitness high and your joint trauma low. Some people like to attach themselves to a solid object and do their deep-water workout in place, while others like moving around in the pool and then returning to the starting location. You might consider the support of an inexpensive noodle or an aqua belt.

If you want to challenge your upper body more, wear aqua gloves; you can even place ankle cuffs on your legs for additional resistance. There's no right or wrong way—just start moving! Try to work out for 20–40 minutes. However, be careful when doing any deep-water routine because drowning is possible. CAUTION: If you can't swim, do NOT try this routine.

WARM-UP

EXERCISE	PAGE	DURATION
Water Walking	52	3–5 minutes
Sideways Walking	53	3–5 minutes
Skipping	54	3–5 minutes

CARDIOVASCULAR CONDITIONING *repeat as desired*

EXERCISE	PAGE	DURATION
Deep-Water Jogging	88	3–5 minutes
Straight-Leg Kicks (deep-water)	90	3–5 minutes
Soccer Kicks (deep-water)	91	3–5 minutes
Cross-Country Skiing (deep-water)	89	3–5 minutes
Deep-Water Sit-Ups	92	3–5 minutes
Twist (deep-water)	93	3–5 minutes
Rock Around the World (deep-water)	94	3–5 minutes

COOLDOWN

EXERCISE	PAGE	DURATION
Water Walking	52	3–5 minutes
Sideways Walking	53	3–5 minutes
Skipping	54	3–5 minutes

Arthritis

The key to exercise for people with arthritis is to maintain range of motion (joint flexibility). The old saying regarding exercise and arthritis is *"motion is lotion."* Water workouts are ideal as therapy because water can minimize the pain and can assist in possible improvement of range of motion. Below is a list of common guidelines for persons with arthritis as suggested by medical doctors and physical therapists.

- Never exercise unless following the advice of a health-care professional.
- Don't over-exercise.
- Don't neglect your medical routine.
- Don't mask pain by over-medicating.
- Don't exercise a "hot joint" (a joint that's swollen or warm to the touch).
- Obey the two-hour rule: If you hurt more two hours post-exercise, you did too much. Do less next time.

Be gentle and start slowly. Perform this workout only as tolerated.

WARM-UP

EXERCISE	PAGE	DURATION
Water Walking	52	as needed or tolerated
Sideways Walking	53	as needed or tolerated

LOWER-BODY CONDITIONING

EXERCISE	PAGE	DURATION
Leg Extension	66	as needed or tolerated
Side Leg Raise	64	as needed or tolerated
Toe Lift	68	as needed or tolerated
1-2-3 Leg Raise & Hold	63	as needed or tolerated

UPPER-BODY CONDITIONING

EXERCISE	PAGE	DURATION
Hula Hands	74	as needed or tolerated
Breaststroke Arms	69	as needed or tolerated
Frontal Raise	58	as needed or tolerated
Arm Curls	75	as needed or tolerated

CARDIOVASCULAR CONDITIONING

EXERCISE	PAGE	DURATION
High Steps with Hula Hands	77 / 74	as needed or tolerated
Cross-Country Skiing with Arm Curls	79 / 75	as needed or tolerated
Leg Curl with Frontal Raise	65 / 58	as needed or tolerated

STRETCHING

EXERCISE	PAGE	DURATION
Calf Stretch	95	as needed or tolerated
Shoulder Stretch	98	as needed or tolerated
Elbow Touches	97	as needed or tolerated
Wrist Stretches	99	as needed or tolerated
Lower Back Stretch	100	as needed or tolerated

Frozen Shoulder

A frozen shoulder usually results from non-use of the shoulder because of a painful shoulder condition such as tendinitis or bursitis. If the arm isn't used for a period of time, adhesions may form on the sleeve-like structure that holds the ball and socket portion of the shoulder joint together. If the shoulder isn't moved for two to three weeks, these adhesions will become very dense and strong and will result in a shoulder that can't move freely—or, frozen shoulder. Water will minimize the pain and possibly improve range of motion. If a shoulder hasn't been used for a long period of time, a health-care professional should be consulted. For more information, see one of my other books, *Healthy Shoulder Handbook* (Ulysses Press, 2010).

Caution: Avoid forceful arm movements or extreme range of motion; move arms slowly through full range of motion under the water.

WARM-UP

EXERCISE	PAGE	DURATION
Sideways Walking	53	as needed or tolerated
Cross-Country Skiing	79	as needed or tolerated

UPPER-BODY CONDITIONING

EXERCISE	PAGE	DURATION
Chest Tap	75	as needed or tolerated
Hula Hands	74	as needed or tolerated
Arm Curls	75	as needed or tolerated
Paddlewheels	74	as needed or tolerated

STRETCHING

EXERCISE	PAGE	DURATION
Elbow Touches	97	as needed or tolerated
Double Wood Chop	98	as needed or tolerated
Shoulder Stretch	98	as needed or tolerated

Low Back Pain

Low back pain is caused by a variety of sources—weak abdominals, tight hamstrings and quadriceps, improper body mechanics, poor posture, overuse, facet and joint problems, and herniated discs. Many arm movements, such as overhead reaching and arm extension, affect the low back. Vertical jumping can also bother those with low back issues. Some water exercisers injure their backs when they do lateral leg raises and lean too much at the waist; the leg should only be raised 45–50 degrees, the toes should point forward, and the trunk should be stabilized and not move.

Exercises that strengthen the abdominals and stretch the hamstrings as well as the low back muscles are recommended. If you have a back problem, good neutral spine technique is especially important. Avoid using leg and ankle weights, as well as hand paddles that cause you to "feel it" in your low back. Here are other tips for a safe workout:

- Keep movements fluid.
- If pain is present more than two hours post-exercise, cut back exercise duration and/or intensity.
- Avoid impact activities.
- Perform exercises in warm water (82–92°F) if possible.
- Try to move through full range of motion and, if possible, keep it pain free.
- Listen to your body.

WARM-UP

EXERCISE	PAGE	DURATION
Water Walking	52	as needed or tolerated
Sideways Walking	53	as needed or tolerated

LOWER-BODY CONDITIONING

EXERCISE	PAGE	DURATION
Leg Extension	66	as needed or tolerated
Side Leg Raise	64	as needed or tolerated
Heel Raise	67	as needed or tolerated

UPPER-BODY CONDITIONING

EXERCISE	PAGE	DURATION
Lateral Raise	57	as needed or tolerated
Chest Tap	59	as needed or tolerated
Fly	56	as needed or tolerated

CARDIOVASCULAR CONDITIONING

EXERCISE	PAGE	DURATION
Deep-Water Jogging	88	as needed or tolerated
Cross-Country Skiing (deep-water)	89	as needed or tolerated

STRETCHING

EXERCISE	PAGE	DURATION
Lower Back Stretch	100	as needed or tolerated
Calf Stretch	95	as needed or tolerated
Hamstring Stretch	95	as needed or tolerated

Hip

Although the hip is the powerhouse of the body, many conditions (from bursitis to arthritis to athletic injuries) can affect the joint. Deep-water exercise is a great way to improve range of motion without inducing trauma.

WARM-UP

EXERCISE	PAGE	DURATION
Water Walking	52	as needed or tolerated
Sideways Walking	53	as needed or tolerated

LOWER-BODY CONDITIONING

EXERCISE	PAGE	DURATION
Forward Leg Raise	61	as needed or tolerated
Leg Curl	65	as needed or tolerated
Deep-Water Jogging	88	as needed or tolerated
Cross-Country Skiing (deep-water)	89	as needed or tolerated

STRETCHING

EXERCISE	PAGE	DURATION
Calf Stretch	95	as needed or tolerated
Lower Back Stretch	100	as needed or tolerated
Hamstring Stretch	95	as needed or tolerated

Knee

If you have knee issues, it's a good idea to keep "soft knees" when doing a water workout. Additionally, avoid twisting your body with your feet planted; the knees and toes should *always* point in the same direction. Performing very wide jumping jacks or jumping and landing without bending the knees to absorb the load can aggravate knee problems. Also, any exercise that uses the quadriceps forcefully, such as leg extensions, can trigger knee pain. Remember: Force rather than speed is better when doing leg exercises. Another precaution is to avoid overflexion of the knee joint when doing quadriceps stretches (i.e., bringing the heel toward the buttocks). Practice learning how to jump and land correctly.

WARM-UP

EXERCISE	PAGE	DURATION
Water Walking	52	as needed or tolerated
Sideways Walking	53	as needed or tolerated

LOWER-BODY CONDITIONING

EXERCISE	PAGE	DURATION
Side Leg Raise	64	as needed or tolerated
Forward Leg Raise	61	as needed or tolerated
Cross-Country Skiing	79	as needed or tolerated
High Steps	77	as needed or tolerated

STRETCHING

EXERCISE	PAGE	DURATION
Calf Stretch	95	as needed or tolerated
Ankle Circles	96	as needed or tolerated

Shin Splints

Shin splints refer to the pain that occurs in the front of the lower leg when the connective tissue pulls away from the bone. Running or aerobic dancing on hard surfaces can contribute to shin splints. Anatomical abnormalities of the foot, as well as strength and flexibility imbalances in the lower leg muscles, can also result in shin splints.

WARM-UP

EXERCISE	PAGE	DURATION
Sideways Walking	53	as needed or tolerated

LOWER-BODY CONDITIONING

EXERCISE	PAGE	DURATION
Heel Raise	67	as needed or tolerated
Toe Lift	68	as needed or tolerated

CARDIOVASCULAR CONDITIONING

EXERCISE	PAGE	DURATION
Deep-Water Jogging	88	as needed or tolerated
Cross-Country Skiing (deep-water)	89	as needed or tolerated

STRETCHING

EXERCISE	PAGE	DURATION
Ankle Circles	96	as needed or tolerated
Calf Stretch	95	as needed or tolerated
Heel Raise	67	as needed or tolerated
Toe Lift	68	as needed or tolerated

Ankle/Feet

Even though injuries to the ankles and feet are greatly reduced in the water, it's important to pay attention to the way you land to avoid supination and pronation problems. There are several ways to lessen the impact on the feet: working in deeper water, wearing aquatic shoes (which also protect the bottoms of the feet), wearing an aqua-jogger while performing suspended deep-water exercises. Use caution with range-of-motion and strengthening moves until any swelling/pain subsides—don't overstretch. Gradually increase weight bearing. People with diabetes need to pay attention to drying their feet completely; consider using a hair dryer to blow-dry between the toes.

WARM-UP

EXERCISE	PAGE	DURATION
Ankle Circles	96	as needed or tolerated
Calf Stretch	95	as needed or tolerated
Water Walking	52	as needed or tolerated
Sideways Walking	53	as needed or tolerated
Forward Leg Raise	61	as needed or tolerated

LOWER-BODY CONDITIONING

EXERCISE	PAGE	DURATION
Heel Raise	67	as needed or tolerated
Toe Lift	68	as needed or tolerated
1-2-3 Leg Raise & Hold	63	as needed or tolerated
Straight-Leg Kicks	80	as needed or tolerated

STRETCHING

EXERCISE	PAGE	DURATION
Calf Stretch	95	as needed or tolerated
Ankle Circles	96	as needed or tolerated

Freeflow Routine 1

This routine is designed for people who like to express their creativity. Basically, select five of your favorite cardiovascular leg moves (pages 77–83) and five of your favorite arm add-ons (pages 69–76).
Then turn on your music or even a clock.

1. Start with one leg move and stay with it for five minutes or switch at the end of every song, but switch your arm motions every minute. One example is to begin with cross-country legs and arm flies, then switch to punching, etc. Then switch to a different leg movement and use the same arm motion.
2. After five songs or 20–25 minutes, grab a noodle and do four songs' worth of deep-water moves.
3. Finish up with some upper-body strength training and a few minutes of stretching.

Freeflow Routine 2

This workout (and my personal favorite) is similar to the first routine, except you need enough space around you to move in every direction. Ten feet in all directions is fine. As with Routine 1, allow your body and your creativity to be the guide. I like to start with jogging forward and backward with breaststroke arms, then switch to cross-country legs with jumping jack arms, etc. It's more challenging to select arm motions that counteract the direction in which you're traveling (e.g., hugging arms and forward jogging). Mix and match to meet your fancy, then try the same concept with deep-water exercises. Turn on some motivating music and go with the flow!

PART 3
The Exercises

Water Walking

target: thermal warm-up

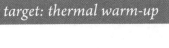

STARTING POSITION: Stand at a comfortable depth in the pool, ideally waist to chest deep.

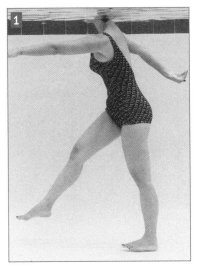

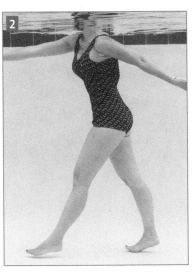

1–2 Walk back and forth across the pool, swinging your arms fully as if walking, then progress to breaststroke arm motions, keeping your arms in the water. Take both large and small strides. Depending on how you feel, you may stop at each end and perform a gentle leg stretch.

VARIATIONS: Walk on your heels. Walk on your toes.

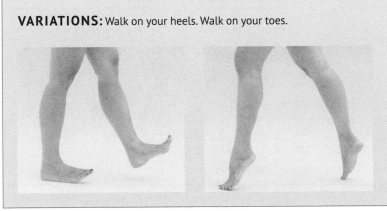

STARTING POSITION: Stand at a comfortable depth in the pool, ideally waist to chest deep.

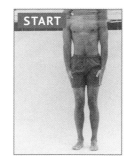
START

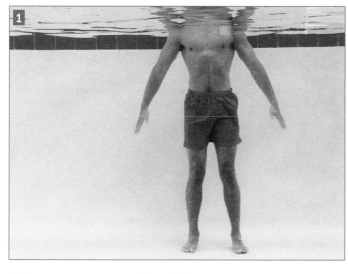
1

1–2 Walk sideways across the pool, using your arms fully to the side while keeping them underwater. Take both large and small steps.

Depending on how you feel, you may stop at each end and perform a gentle leg stretch.

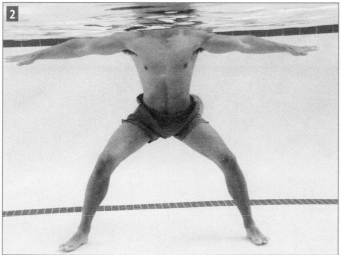
2

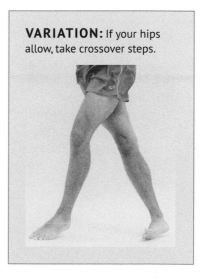
VARIATION: If your hips allow, take crossover steps.

Skipping

target: thermal warm-up

STARTING POSITION: Stand at a comfortable depth in the pool, ideally waist to chest deep.

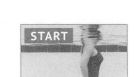

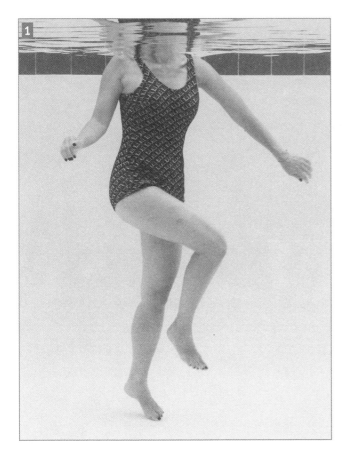

1 Skip across the pool. Use your arms any way you want to loosen up your body.

Now hop, skip, and jump across the pool.

Chest Press
target: chest, shoulders, upper back

STARTING POSITION: Stand tall in a stable position (e.g., one leg forward, one leg back) and hold a VRTD in each hand at your chest, VRTD facing forward.

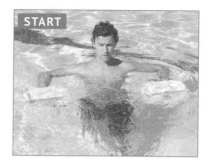
START

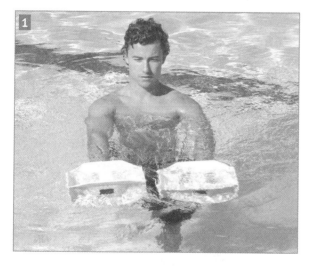
1

1 Push both arms forward as quickly as possible.

2 Return to starting position.

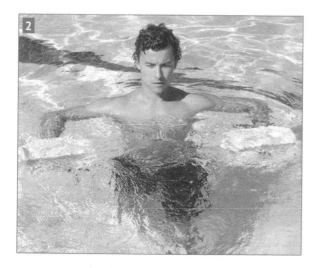
2

VARIATION: You can also do this one arm at a time.

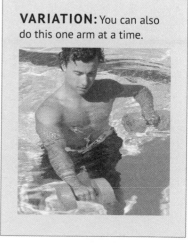

Fly

STARTING POSITION: Stand tall in a stable position (e.g., one leg forward, one leg back) and hold a VRTD in each hand. Extend both arms in front of your shoulders, palms facing each other.

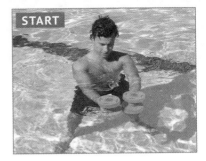

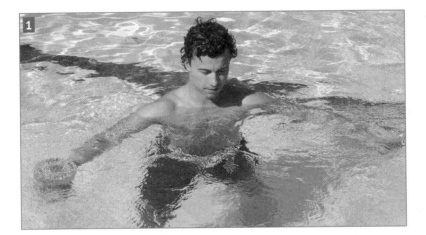

1 As quickly as possible, take your arms out to the sides.

2 Return to starting position.

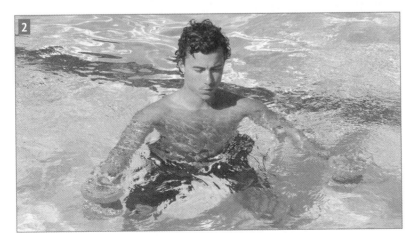

Lateral Raise

STARTING POSITION: Stand tall in a stable position (e.g., one leg forward, one leg back) and hold a VRTD in each hand, arms along your sides.

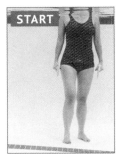

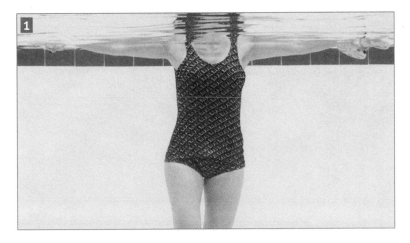

1 Lift both arms up sideways to surface level as quickly as possible.

2 Return to starting position.

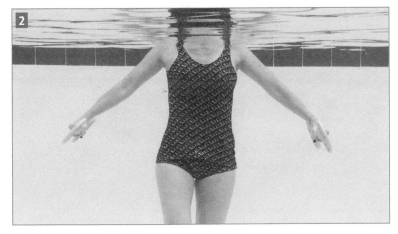

VARIATION: You can also do this one arm at a time.

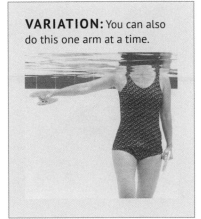

Frontal Raise

target: shoulders (frontal aspect)

STARTING POSITION: Stand tall in a stable position (e.g., one leg forward, one leg back) and hold a VRTD in each hand, arms out in front of you at shoulder height and palms facing down.

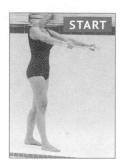

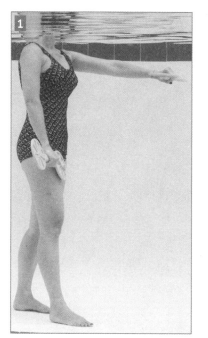

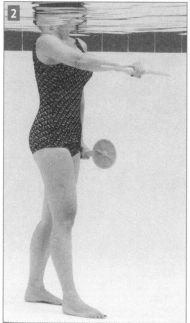

1 Push your right arm down to your thigh/hip area.

2 Bring it up to surface level as quickly as possible; when your right arm comes up, push your left arm down.

Continue alternating arms.

STARTING POSITION: Stand tall in a stable position (e.g., one leg forward, one leg back) and hold a VRTD in each hand with your arms extended out to the sides at shoulder level, palms facing forward.

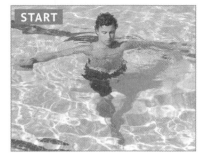

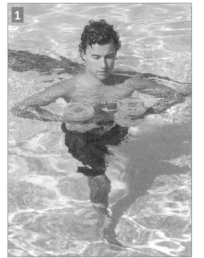 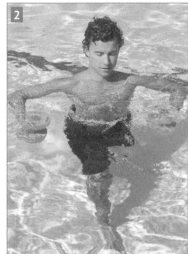

1 As quickly as possible, bend your elbows and bring your hands to your chest.

2 Return to starting position.

VARIATION: You can also do this one arm at a time.

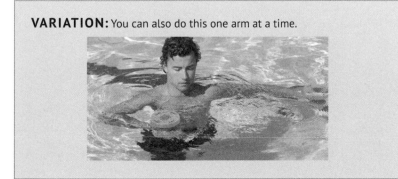

Washboard

target: biceps, triceps, trapezius, shoulders

STARTING POSITION: Stand tall but lean slightly forward. Hold a VRTD in each hand near your armpits.

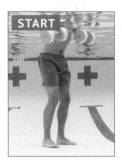
START

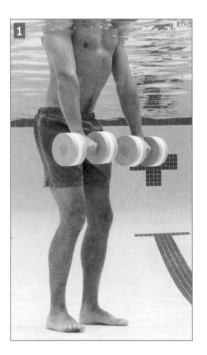

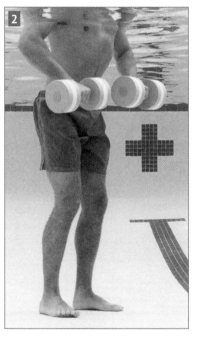

1–2 Press both arms down and up vigorously.

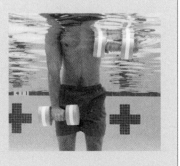

PISTON ARMS VARIATION:
As you advance, you can move one arm down as the other arm comes up.

Forward Leg Raise

target: quadriceps

STARTING POSITION: Stand tall with proper neutral posture. You may place your hands on your hips.

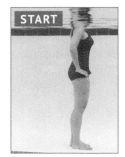

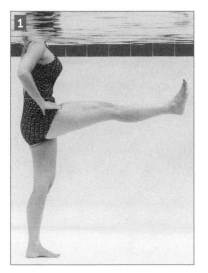

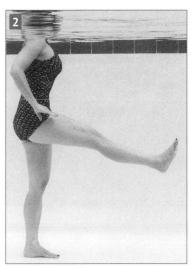

1 Keeping your right leg straight, quickly lift it straight up with your toes pointed up. You should feel this motion in your quads.

2 Keeping your lower back motionless, quickly lower your leg.

Finish your reps on this leg and then perform with your left leg.

Backward Leg Raise

target: gluteal region

Caution: If you have lower back issues, be careful not to arch your back when performing this exercise.

STARTING POSITION: Stand tall with proper neutral posture. You may place your hands on your hips.

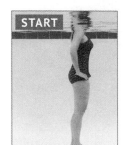

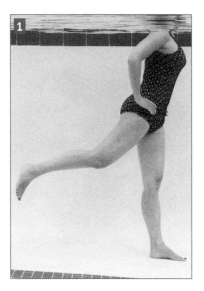

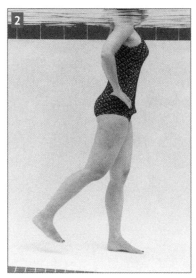

1 Keeping your right leg straight, slowly swing it backward, being mindful to engage your butt muscles.

2 Smoothly return to starting position.

Finish your reps on this leg and then perform with your left leg.

1-2-3 Leg Raise & Hold

target: quadriceps, hamstrings, glutes

This exercise combines the movements of the Forward Leg Raise and Backward Leg Raise.

STARTING POSITION: Stand tall with proper neutral posture. You may place your hands on your hips.

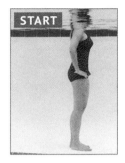

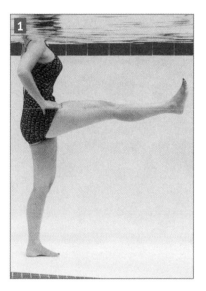

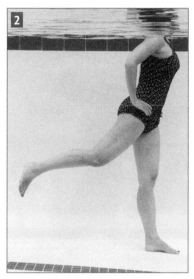

1 Keeping your right leg straight, quickly swing your leg forward with your toes pointed up. You should feel this motion in your quads.

2 Keeping your lower back motionless, quickly swing your leg backward.

Now swing it forward again and hold the position for a few seconds. Continue swinging, holding the position of the third swing. After you've performed the prescribed number of reps, switch legs.

Side Leg Raise

target: inner and outer thighs

CAUTION: Be careful if you have hip issues.

STARTING POSITION: Stand tall with proper neutral posture.

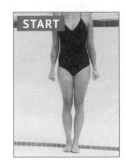

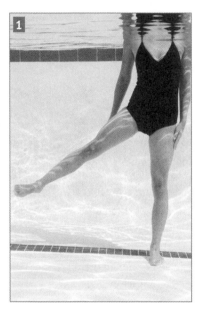

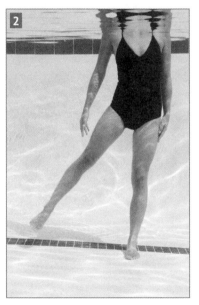

1 Keeping your right leg straight, quickly lift it out to the side. Be mindful that the motion comes from the hip joint; don't swing your leg or lean forward.

2 Quickly and smoothly return to starting position.

Finish your reps on this leg and then perform with your left leg.

Leg Curl

You may want to perform a hamstring stretch between sets to avoid cramps.
CAUTION: If you have lower back issues, be careful to not arch your lower back.

STARTING POSITION: Stand tall with proper neutral posture.

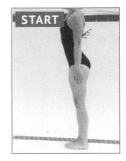

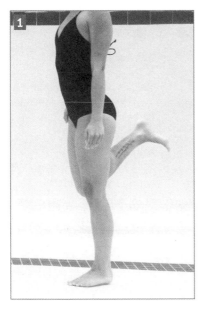

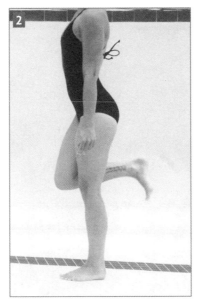

1 Keeping your foot flexed, bend your right knee to bring your right heel toward your butt as high as is comfortable.

2 Straighten your leg again.

Finish your reps on this leg and then perform with your left leg.

Leg Extension

target: quadriceps, hamstrings

CAUTION: Be careful not to snap the knee joint nor hyperextend the knee.

STARTING POSITION: Stand tall with proper neutral posture and place your hands on your hips.

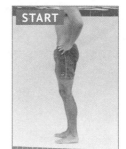

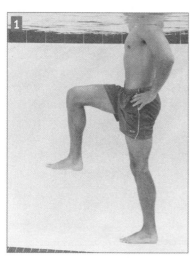

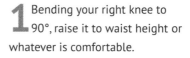

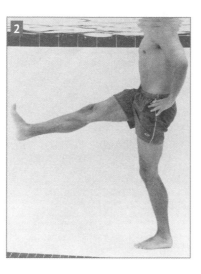

1 Bending your right knee to 90°, raise it to waist height or whatever is comfortable.

2 Extend your leg straight out, but don't force the motion.

3 Curl your leg back to the starting position.

Finish your reps on this leg and then perform with your left leg.

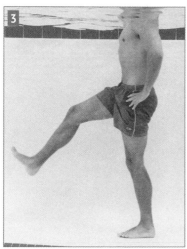

Heel Raise

CAUTION: Stay mindful of cramps. It's recommended that you stretch the calf muscles between sets.

STARTING POSITION: Stand tall with proper neutral posture and your feet together.

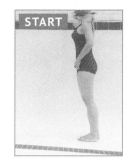

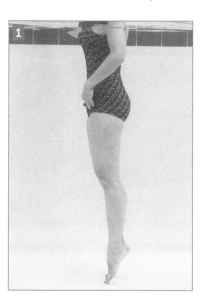

1 Keeping your feet together, come up on the balls of your feet.

Lower to starting position.

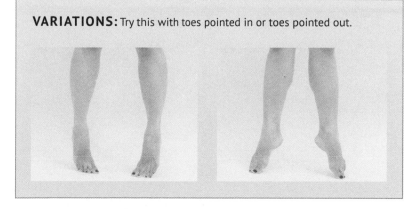

VARIATIONS: Try this with toes pointed in or toes pointed out.

67

Toe Lift

target: shins

This exercise is excellent for people who have foot drop and bouts of shin splints.

STARTING POSITION: Stand tall with proper neutral posture.

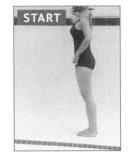

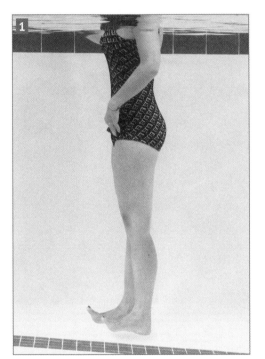

1 Slowly rock back onto your heels, lifting the fronts of your feet off the pool floor. Hold for several seconds.

Lower to starting position.

Cardiovascular Conditioning

This cardiovascular section is arranged menu style, allowing you to mix and match upper-body motions with different lower-body movements for an endless variety of exercises. Generally when I teach a class, I have the class do the same leg motions for about five minutes and change the arm motions every minute. This approach keeps the exercise from getting monotonous and prevents muscle fatigue. For a full 40-minute workout, start with high steps (page 77) and move through the leg movements, ending with the jumping sequence. The goal is to do each movement for five minutes at the intensity of your choice. When you get to the jumping sequence, do each jump for one minute. Each movement includes recommended arm variations; you can do these or pick others from the arm add-ons menu (pages 69–76). For a quick warm-up, pick any of the lower-body movements (pages 77–83) and pair it with a few upper-body motions.

ARM ADD-ONS

Breaststroke Arms *target: upper back*

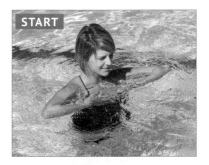 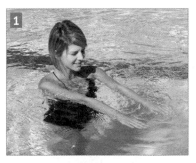 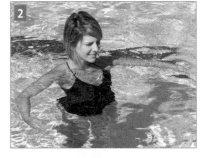

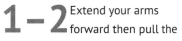

STARTING POSITION: Hold your hands at your chest.

1–2 Extend your arms forward then pull the water into your sides as if doing a breaststroke.

Hug Arms

target: *biceps*

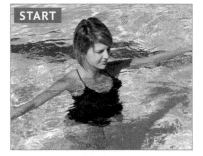

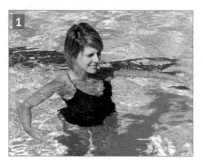

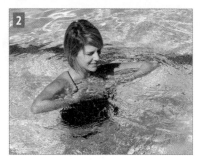

STARTING POSITION: Raise your arms to shoulder height and bring them out to the sides so that they're parallel to the floor.

1–2 Scoop your arms in toward your chest as if hugging someone.

Continue scooping water in toward your chest.

Washboard Arms

target: *biceps, triceps, trapezius, shoulders*

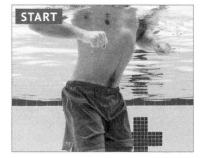

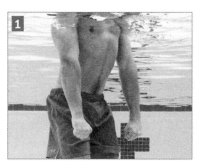

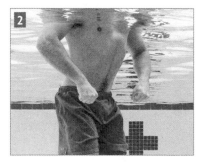

STARTING POSITION: Hold your hands near your armpits.

1–2 Press both arms down and up vigorously.

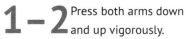

Piston Arms

target: biceps, triceps, trapezius, shoulders

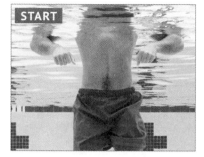 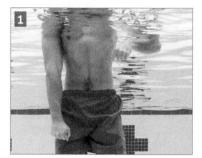 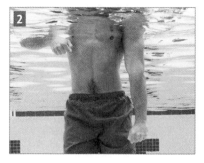

STARTING POSITION: Hold your hands near your armpits.

1–2 Press your right arm down. As you bring your right arm up, simultaneously press your left arm down.

Fly Arms

target: chest, upper back

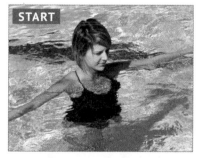 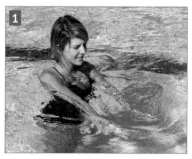

STARTING POSITION: Extend your arms straight out to the sides at shoulder height.

1 Keeping your arms straight, clap your hands together quickly in front of your body.

Return to starting position.

Punching

target: triceps, shoulders, chest

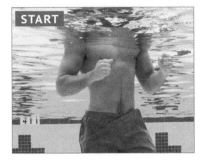

STARTING POSITION: Hold your hands at your chest.

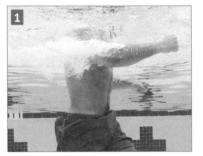

1–2 Extend one arm forward then bring it

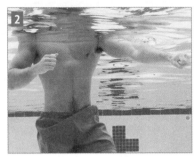

back to your chest as the other arm punches forward.

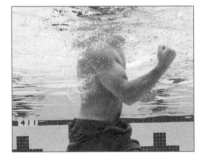

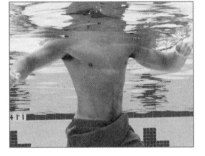

3–4 You can also perform uppercuts, roundhouses, or jabs.

VARIATION: Punch with both arms simultaneously. For additional cardio work, punch with vigor.

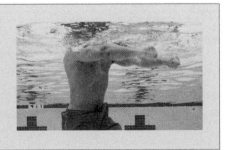

Arm Circles

target: shoulders, upper back

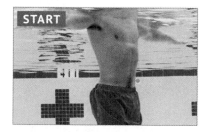 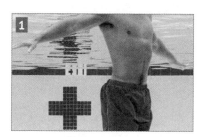 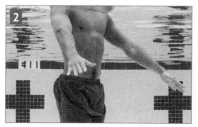

STARTING POSITION: Extend your arms straight out to the sides at shoulder height, keeping them underwater.

1–2 Keeping your arms straight, make small circles forward then progress to larger and faster arm circles.

Reverse direction.

Cross-Country Arms

target: shoulders

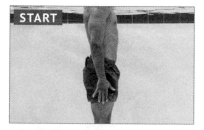 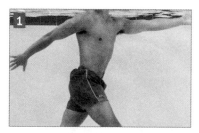 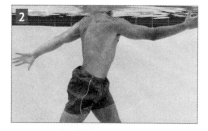

STARTING POSITION: Rest your arms along your sides.

1–2 Keeping your arms somewhat straight, pump your arms back and forth as if you had a ski pole in each hand. One arm should move forward as the other moves backward.

To increase resistance, cup your hands. To decrease resistance, slice through the water.

Paddlewheels

target: upper body

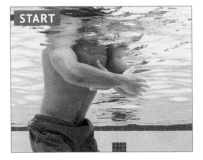

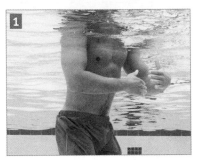

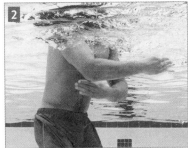

STARTING POSITION: Bend your arms 90 degrees with your arms in front of your chest approximately shoulder height.

1–2 Moving only from your elbows, circle your arms forward.

Reverse direction.

Hula Hands

target: upper body

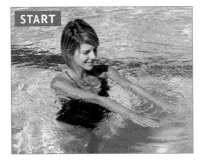

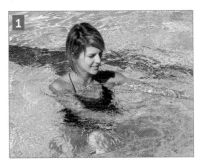

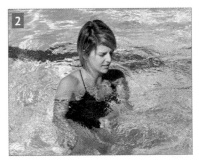

STARTING POSITION: Extend your arms straight out in front of you at shoulder height.

1–2 Move your arms and hands as if you're doing a hula dance, keeping your arms straight but soft. Be creative

with the arm motions—notice the difference in resistance.

Chest Tap Arms

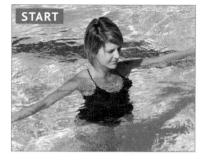

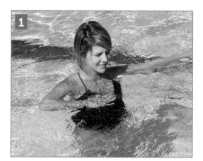

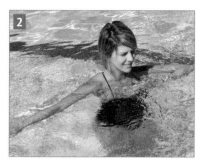

STARTING POSITION: Extend your arms straight out to the sides at shoulder height.

1–2 Bending your arms at the elbow, tap yourself on the chest, alternating hands.

Arm Curls

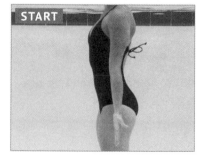

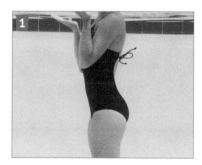

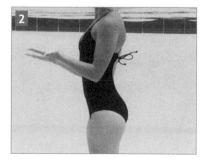

STARTING POSITION: Rest your arms along your sides.

1 With open hands, bring your right hand toward your right shoulder and your left hand toward your left shoulder.

2 Lower your arms and repeat quickly.

Jumping Jack Arms: Side

target: shoulders (lateral)

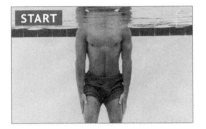

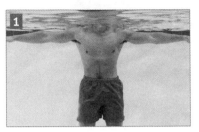

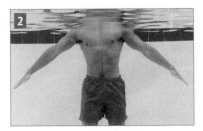

STARTING POSITION: Rest your arms along your sides.

1–2 Keeping your arms straight, quickly lift your arms sideways to the surface of the water. Keep your arms underwater—you get the resistance from the water, not the air.

Quickly return to starting position and repeat.

Jumping Jack Arms: Frontal

target: shoulders (frontal)

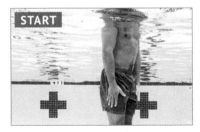

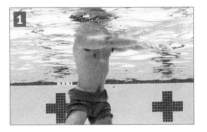

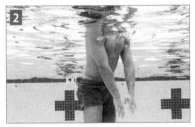

STARTING POSITION: Rest your arms along your sides.

1–2 Keeping your arms straight, quickly lift them forward to the surface of the water. Keep your arms underwater—you get the resistance from the water, not the air.

Quickly return to starting position and repeat.

VARIATION: You can do this one arm at a time. Raise one arm to the surface of the water; as you lower the raised arm, simultaneously bring the other one up.

High Steps

target: aerobic fitness, total leg endurance

Perform leg movements for five minutes; change arm movements every 60 seconds.

STARTING POSITION: Stand tall with proper neutral posture.

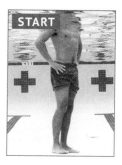

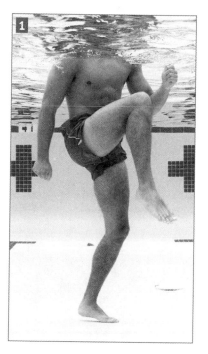

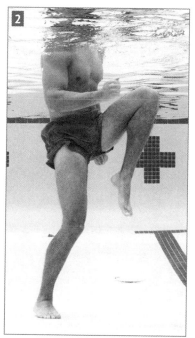

1–2 Lift your knees high as if stepping on a chair; try to get your heels to the pool floor periodically to avoid calf cramps. Add arms (see variations below) as desired.

RECOMMENDED ARM VARIATIONS: Punching (page 72), Paddlewheels (page 74).

Jumping Jacks

target: aerobic fitness, inner/outer leg endurance

Perform leg movements for five minutes; change arm movements every 60 seconds.

STARTING POSITION: Stand tall with your feet together and arms by your sides.

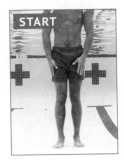

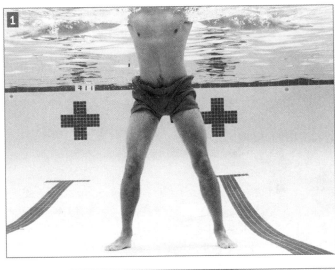

1 Jump up and spread your legs a comfortable distance, approximately shoulder-width apart. Add arms (see variations below) as desired.

2 Return your legs to starting position and continue jumping.

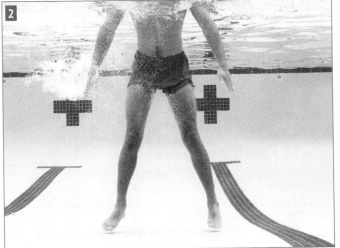

RECOMMENDED ARM VARIATIONS: Jumping Jack Arms: Side (page 76), Jumping Jack Arms: Frontal (page 76), Fly Arms (page 71).

Cross-Country Skiing

target: aerobic fitness, total leg endurance

Perform leg movements for five minutes; change arm movements every 60 seconds. CAUTION: Be careful not to lunge farther than is comfortable as this could trigger lower back pain and knee discomfort.

STARTING POSITION: Stand tall with your arms along your sides.

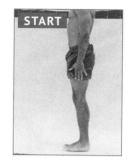
START

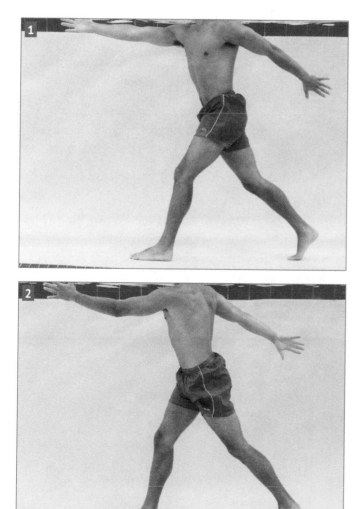

1 Jump up and move one leg forward and the other leg backward a comfortable distance. Add arms (see variations below) as desired.

2 Continue alternating leg motions.

RECOMMENDED ARM VARIATIONS: Breaststroke Arms (page 69), Cross-Country Arms (page 73), Arm Curls (page 75).

79

LEG MOVEMENTS

Straight-Leg Kicks

target: quadriceps, hamstrings

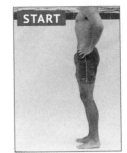
START

Perform leg movements for five minutes; change arm movements every 60 seconds.

STARTING POSITION: Stand tall with your hands on your hips.

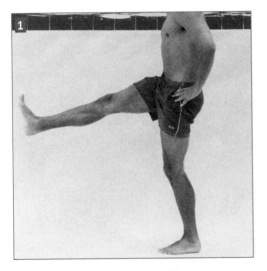

1 Quickly lift your right leg straight up to the front; be careful not to kick too high. Add arms (see variations below) as desired.

2 Alternating quickly, bring your right leg down and lift your left.

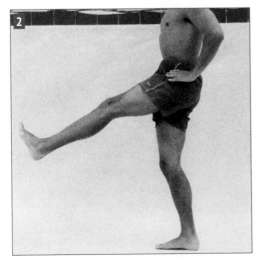

RECOMMENDED ARM VARIATIONS: Jumping Jack Arms: Side (page 76), right hand to left leg and vice versa .

Soccer Kicks

target: quadriceps, hamstrings

Perform leg movements for five minutes; change arm movements every 60 seconds.

STARTING POSITION: Stand tall with your hands on your hips.

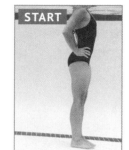

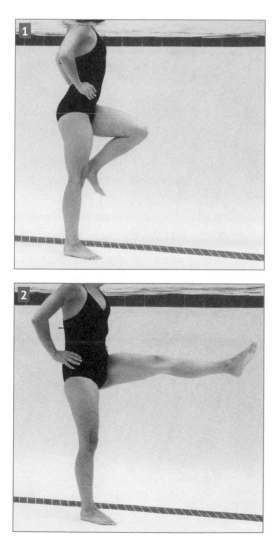

1–2 Lift your right knee and extend your leg as if kicking someone in the rear; be careful not to lock out your knee or kick too high. Add arms (see variations below) as desired.

Bring your leg down and quickly kick with the other leg.

RECOMMENDED ARM VARIATIONS: Chest Tap Arms (page 75), Arm Circles (page 73).

Butt Kickers

target: aerobic fitness, hamstrings

Perform leg movements for five minutes; change arm movements every 60 seconds. CAUTION: People with knee issues should only bend to 90°.

STARTING POSITION: Stand tall with your arms alongside your body.

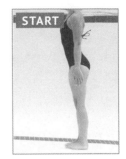

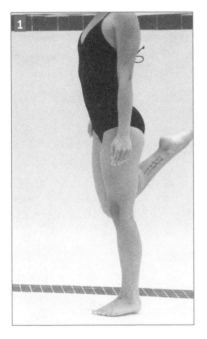

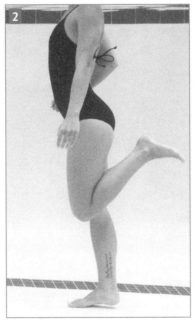

1 Flex/curl your right leg toward your bottom. Be careful not to curl your leg too high or you might get a hamstring cramp.

2 Return to starting position and perform with your left leg.

Continue alternating legs, adding arms (see variations below) as desired.

RECOMMENDED ARM VARIATIONS: Arm Curls (page 75), Fly Arms (page 71).

Rocking Horse

target: aerobic cool down, overall body toning

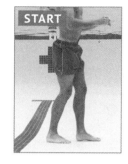

Perform leg movements for five minutes; change arm movements every 60 seconds.

STARTING POSITION: Stand tall with your left leg forward and right leg back.

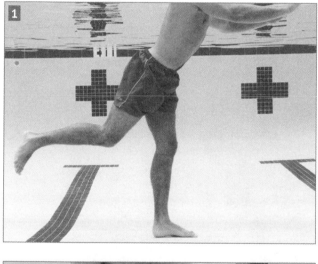

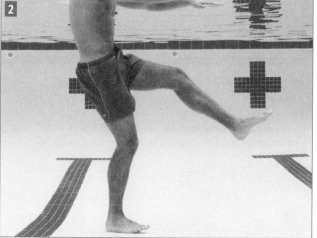

1–2 Rock forward onto your left leg then immediately rock back to your right leg—the movement should be fluid and smooth. Add arms (see variations below) as desired.

Continue rocking back and forth for one minute then move the right leg to the forward position.

RECOMMENDED ARM VARIATIONS: Breaststroke Arms (page 69), Hug Arms (page 70), Jumping Jack Arms: Side (page 76).

Underwater Rockets

target: aerobic fitness, leg power

STARTING POSITION: Stand with your shoulders under the water, knees slightly bent.

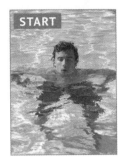

START

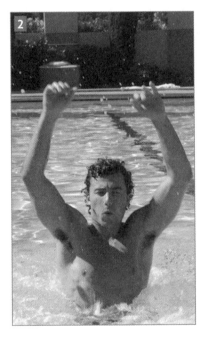

1–2 Jump up and down as high as you can for one minute.

STARTING POSITION: Stand with proper neutral posture, knees slightly bent. You can place your hands on your hips if you like. Imagine you're at the 6 o'clock position of a clock.

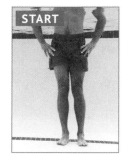

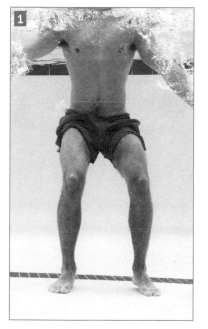

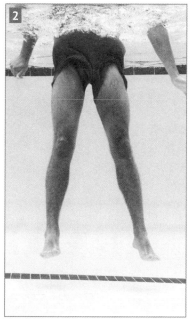

1–2 Jump forward to 12 o'clock (you decide how far forward to jump). Without pausing, jump back to 6 o'clock.

Continue for one minute.

RECOMMENDED ARM VARIATIONS: Breaststroke Arms (page 69) as you pull forward, Hug Arms (page 70) as you go back, Jumping Jack Arms to the front and sides (page 76)

9 O'clock to 3 O'clock Jumps

target: aerobic fitness, leg power

STARTING POSITION: Stand tall with proper neutral posture and place your hands on your hips. Imagine you're at the 9 o'clock position of a clock.

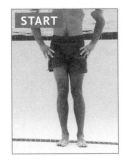

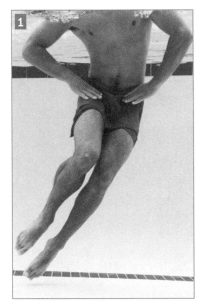

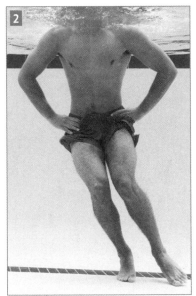

1–2 Jump over to 3 o'clock (you decide how far sideward to jump). Without pausing, jump back to 9 o'clock.

Continue for 1 minute.

RECOMMENDED ARM VARIATIONS: Jumping Jack Arms: Side (page 76), Chest Tap Arms (page 75), Arm Curls (page 75).

Jump Rope

target: aerobic fitness, leg endurance

STARTING POSITION: Stand tall with your arms by your sides and hands in fists.

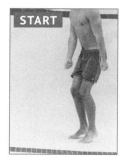

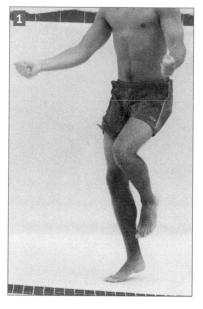

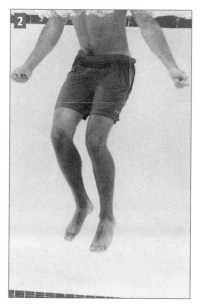

1 Pretend to skip rope by alternating one leg then the other.

Continue for one minute.

2 Pretend to jump rope with both feet together, jumping as high as you want.

Continue for one minute.

Deep-Water Jogging

target: aerobic fitness, total body exercise

STARTING POSITION: With your feet off the bottom of the pool with or without a flotation device and with or without a tethered attachment, lean slightly forward.

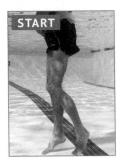
START

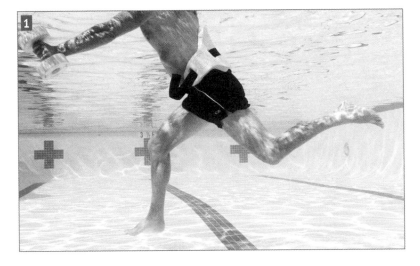

1–2 Move your legs as if jogging and pump your arms as follows:

• Really pump your arms as if running up a hill.

• Punch one arm forward at a time and really recoil it back.

• Perform arm curls.

• Be creative—move your arms any way you wish.

• If you're untethered, use your arm motions to allow you to move a few feet forward and then return to starting position.

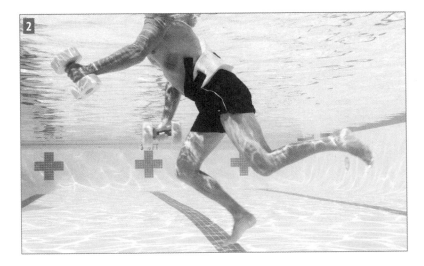

Cross-Country Skiing

target: aerobic fitness, front/rear upper legs

STARTING POSITION: With your feet off the bottom of the pool with or without a flotation device and with or without a tethered attachment, lean slightly forward. Note: An aqua belt can be worn around the midsection for support, or aqua bells can be placed under the armpits or held in each hand with the arms held to the side.

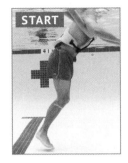

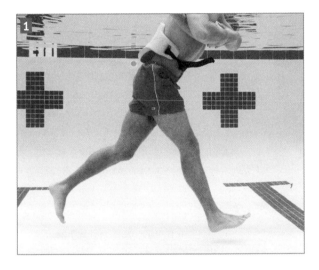

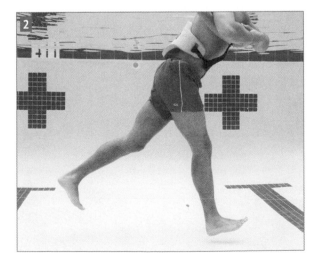

1–2 Keeping your legs fairly straight, slide them forward and backward as if cross-country skiing. The back leg should move back a comfortable distance—do not overstride.

You can also move your arms as follows:

- Pump your arms vigorously to obtain the intensity you desire.

- Punch both arms forward and really recoil them back.

- Act as if you're doing the crawl stroke but keep your arms underwater and pull your hand back as far as possible.

- Perform the breaststroke, pulling your arms hard.

- If you're untethered, use your arm motions to allow you to move a few feet forward and then return to starting position.

89

Straight-Leg Kicks

target: quadriceps

STARTING POSITION: With your feet off the bottom of the pool, with or without a flotation device and with or without a tethered attachment, try to stay somewhat vertical.

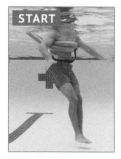

START

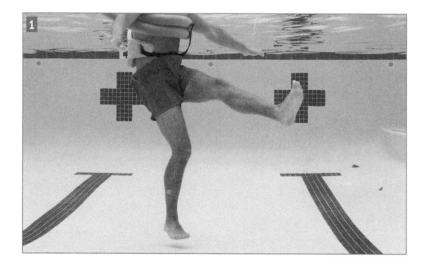

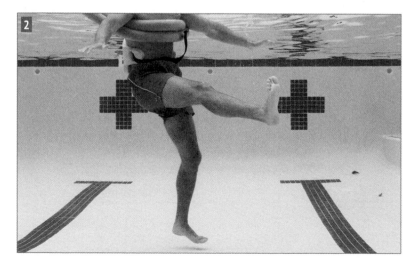

1–2 Keeping your legs straight, alternate swinging your legs forward as if you were a drum majorette. As you do so, move your arms as follows:

• Perform flies.

• Open your arms to the side then clap your hands to your chest (chest taps).

• Combine the flies with chest taps, alternating between the two.

• Combine breaststroke arms and hug arms.

• If you're untethered, use your arm motions to allow you to move a few feet forward and then return to starting position.

STARTING POSITION: With your feet off the bottom of the pool, with or without a flotation device and with or without a tethered attachment, try to stay somewhat vertical.

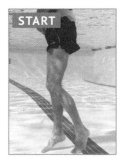
START

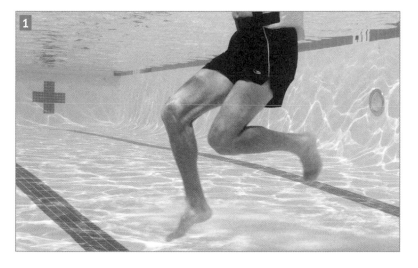

1–2 Move your legs as if you were kicking someone in front of you. As you do so, move your arms as follows:

• Punch your left arm forward as your left leg kicks, then alternate.

• Bring your right hand to your left knee.

• Move your arms as if you're doing the hula.

• Be creative and invent an arm motion that goes with the movement, your mood, or the music.

• If you're untethered, use your arm motions to allow you to move a few feet forward and then return to starting position.

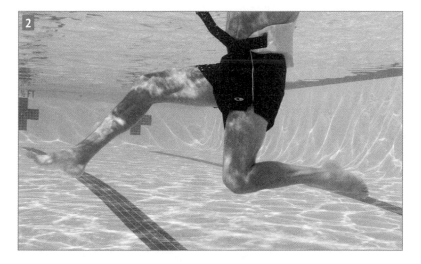

Deep-Water Sit-Ups

target: midsection

These aren't as good as floor sit-ups but they're a lot more fun. Focus on using your abdominal muscles. Many people like to do this exercise with a noodle under their armpits.

STARTING POSITION: With your feet off the bottom of the pool, either with or without a flotation device, lie on your back.

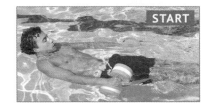

START

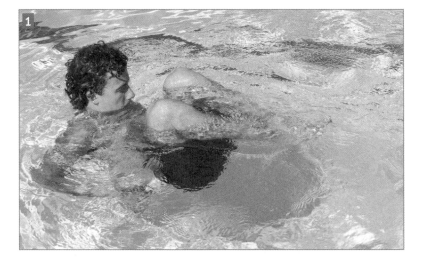

1 Bring your knees to your chest.

2 Extend your legs forward.

Repeat until you can't maintain proper form.

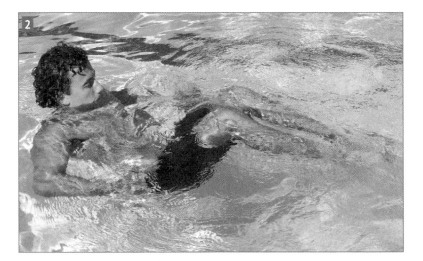

Twist

CAUTION: If you have lower back issues, be extra careful.

STARTING POSITION: With your feet off the bottom of the pool, either with or without a flotation device, lie on your back.

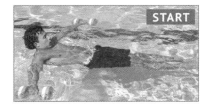
START

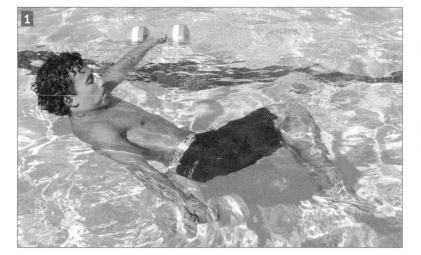
1

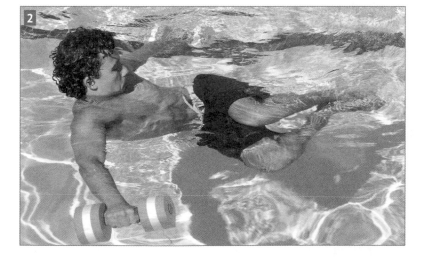
2

1 Bending your knees slightly, move your legs slightly to the left.

2 Return to center and move your legs slightly to the right.

Repeat until you can't maintain proper form.

93

Rock Around the World

target: midsection, butt

CAUTION: *If you have lower back issues, be extra careful.*

STARTING POSITION: With your feet off the bottom of the pool, either with or without a flotation device, lie on your back.

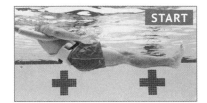

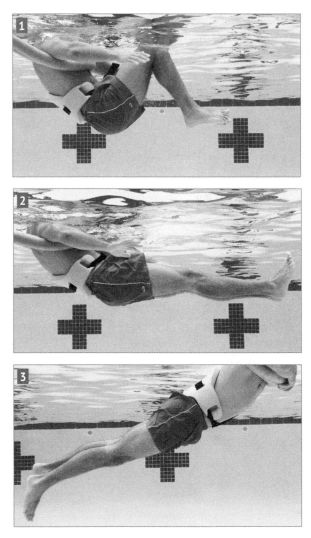

1 Bring your knees to your chest.

2 Extend your legs forward.

3 Pull your legs back in and extend them behind you.

Hamstring Stretch

target: hamstrings

THE STRETCH: Stand either with your back to the wall or unsupported in the water. Grasp one leg with both hands and pull your leg up. Straighten your leg, extend it forward and keep your toes pointed up. This stretch should be felt in the back of the thigh. Hold for 15–30 seconds.

Lower your leg back to starting position. Repeat with your other leg.

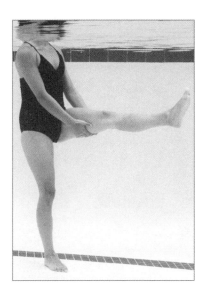

VARIATION: If you have trouble balancing, you can place your foot (toes up) on the wall.

Calf Stretch

target: calves

THE STRETCH: Place one hand on the wall for support. While keeping your heel down, slide your right leg straight back as far as possible. Bend your left knee slightly until the desired stretch is felt in your right calf muscle. Hold for 15–30 seconds.

Repeat on the other leg.

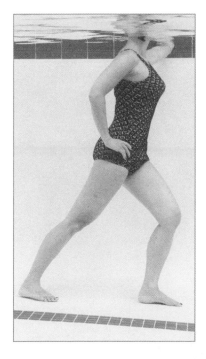

VARIATION: You can also do this by facing a wall and placing both hands on it for support.

Ankle Circles

target: ankle flexibility

STARTING POSITION: Stand either with your back to the wall or unsupported in the water.

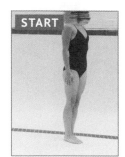

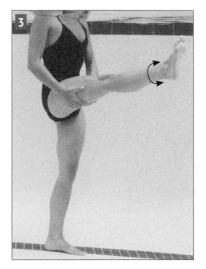

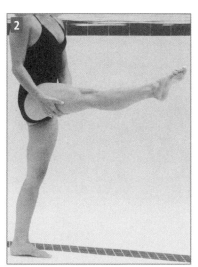

1 Grasp your right leg with both hands and pull your leg up. Keeping your leg straight, extend it forward and keep your toes pointed up. This stretch should be felt in the back of the thigh.

2 While keeping your leg stationary, point your foot forward and then pull it back several times. This motion will improve the range of motion of your ankle joint.

3 While keeping your leg stationary, draw circles in both directions with your foot.

Lower your leg back to starting position and repeat the sequence with your other leg.

STARTING POSITION: Stand tall with proper posture and place your right hand on your right shoulder and your left hand on your left shoulder.

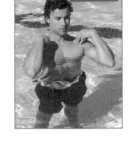

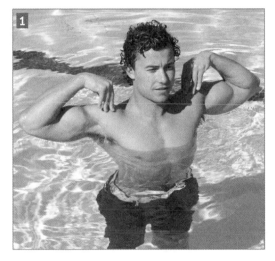

1 Keeping your hands in place, slowly take your elbows out to the sides as far as is comfortable. Hold for 5–15 seconds. Focus on squeezing your shoulder blades together and opening up your chest.

2 Bring your elbows together.

Repeat.

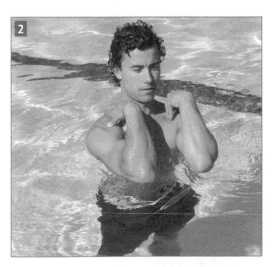

Double Wood Chop
target: shoulders, chest

STARTING POSITION: Stand tall with proper neutral posture. Interlace your fingers in front of your body.

1 Inhale deeply through your nose while slowly lifting your arms as high as possible. Hold for 5–10 seconds.

Slowly lower your arms to starting position.

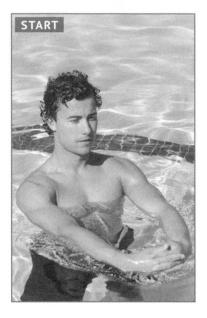 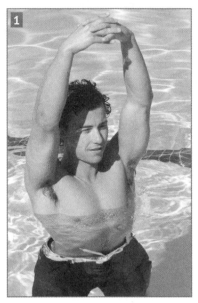

Shoulder Stretch
target: shoulders

THE STRETCH: Stand tall with your feet comfortably apart. Take your right arm across your chest. Place your left hand just above your right elbow and gently press your elbow toward your throat. Hold for 5–10 seconds.

Repeat on the other side.

Wrist Stretch 1

THE STRETCH: Stand tall with proper posture. Extend one arm in front of you at shoulder height, with your palm facing forward and fingers pointing up. With your other hand, gently pull your fingers back until the desired stretch is felt under your wrist. Hold for 10–15 seconds. Repeat on the other arm.

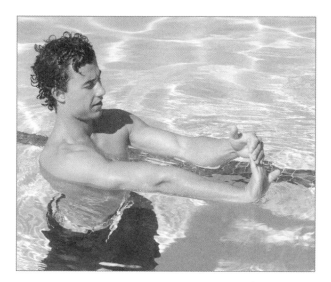

Wrist Stretch 2

THE STRETCH: Extend one arm in front of you at shoulder height, with your palm facing forward and fingers pointing down. With your other hand, gently pull your fingers back until the desired stretch is felt around your wrist. Hold for 10–15 seconds. Repeat on the other arm.

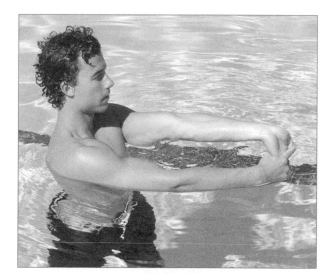

Lower Back Stretch

THE STRETCH: Stand with your back to the wall or unsupported in the water. Grasp one leg with both hands and bring your leg up to your chest. If it feels better, you can round your back. This movement should be felt in your lower back. Hold for 15–30 seconds.

Lower your leg to starting position and repeat with your other leg.

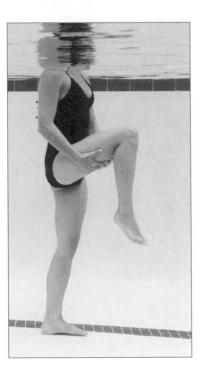

Exercises Index

a

Advanced general conditioning workout, sample, 35–36
Ankle Circles, 96
Ankle/feet workout, sample, 49
Arm add-ons, 69–76
Arm Circles, 73
Arm Curls, 75
Arthritis workout, sample, 41–42

b

Backward Leg Raise, 62
Breaststroke Arms, 69
Butt Kickers, 82

c

Calf Stretch, 95
Cardiovascular conditioning, 69–87; arm add-ons, 69–76; jumping exercises, 84–87; leg movements, 77–83
Chest Press, 55
Chest Tap Arms, 75
Chest Tap, 59
Cross-Country Arms, 73
Cross-Country Skiing, 79
Cross-Country Skiing, Deep-Water, 89

d

Deep-water exercises, 88–94
Deep-Water Jogging, 88
Deep-Water Sit-Ups, 92
Deep-water workout, sample, 39–40
Double Wood Chop, 98

e

Elbow Touches, 97
Exercises, 51–100; cardiovascular, 69–87; deep water, 88–94; lower body, 61–68; stretches, 95–100; upper body, 55–60; warm-ups, 52–54

f

Fly Arms, 71
Fly, 56
Forward Leg Raise, 61
Freeflow routines, 50
Frontal Raise, 58
Frozen shoulder workout, sample, 43

g

General fitness workout, sample, 33–34

h

Hamstring Stretch, 95
Heel Raise, 67
High Steps, 77
Hip workout, sample, 46
Hug Arms, 70
Hula Hands, 74

j

Jump Rope, 87
Jumping exercises, 84–87
Jumping Jack Arms: frontal, 76; side, 76
Jumping Jacks, 78

k

Knee workout, sample, 47

l

Lateral Raise, 57
Leg Curl, 65
Leg Extension, 66
Leg movements, 77–83
Low back pain workout, sample, 44–45
Lower Back Stretch, 100
Lower-body exercises, 61–68

n

9 o'clock to 3 o'clock Jumps, 86

o

1-2-3 Leg Raise & Hold, 63

p

Paddlewheels, 74
Piston Arms, 71
Punching, 72

r

Rock Around the World, 94
Rocking Horse, 83

s

Sample workouts, 32–50
Shin splints workout, sample, 48
Side Leg Raise, 64
Sideways Walking, 53
6 o'clock to 12 o'clock Jumps, 85
Skipping, 54
Soccer Kicks, 81
Soccer Kicks, Deep-Water, 91
Sports conditioning workout,
    sample, 37–38
Straight-Leg Kicks, 80
Straight-Leg Kicks, Deep-Water,
    90
Stretches, 95–100

t

Toe Lift, 68
Twist, 93

u

Underwater Rockets, 84
Upper-body exercises, 55–60

w

Warm-up exercises, 52–54
Washboard Arms, 70
Washboard, 60
Water Walking, 52
Workouts, sample, 32–50
Wrist stretches, 99

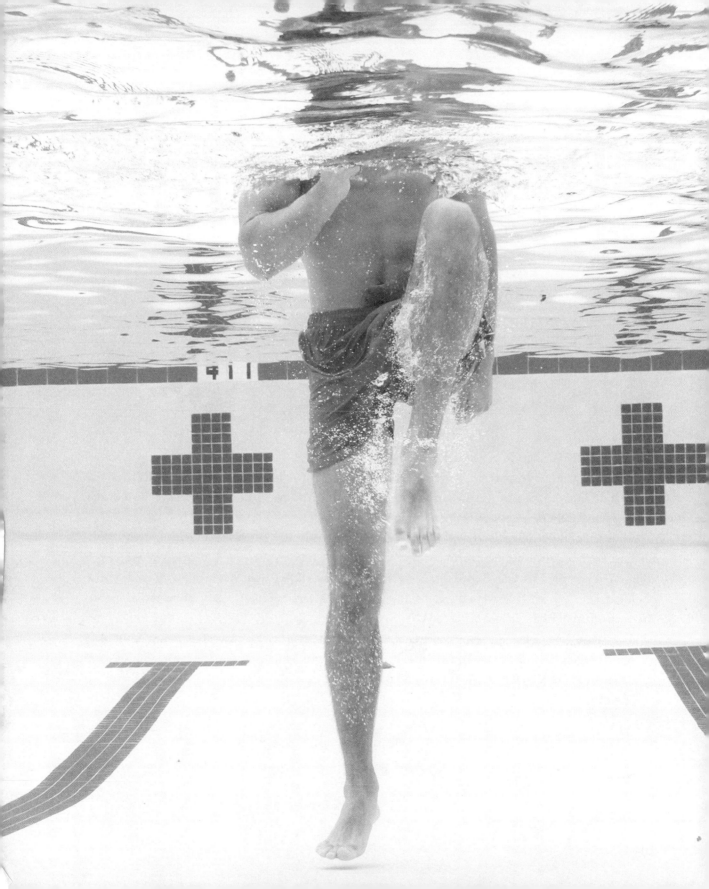

Acknowledgments

This book would not have been possible without the expertise of Lily Chou and Claire Chun. Thanks to my models Sasha Wozniak, Kitty Chiu, and Chris Knopf. Chris also provided insight into some of the water routines included in this book. A special thanks goes to Nancy Kao, executive director of the Forum at Rancho San Antonio, for allowing us the use of their magnificent facilities.

About the Author

DR. KARL KNOPF, author of *Foam Roller Workbook, Healthy Hips Handbook, Healthy Shoulder Handbook, Stretching for 50+, and Weights for 50+*, has been involved in the health and fitness of older adults and the disabled for more than forty years. During this time he has worked in almost every aspect of the industry, from personal training and therapy to consultation.

While at Foothill College, Karl was the coordinator of the Adaptive Fitness Technician Program and Lifelong Learning Institute. He taught disabled students and undergraduates about corrective exercise. In addition to teaching, Karl developed the "Fitness Educators of Older Adults Association" to guide trainers of older adults. Currently Karl is a director at the International Sports Science Association and is on the advisory board of PBS's *Sit and Be Fit* show.

In his spare time he has spoken at conferences, authored many articles, and written numerous books on topics ranging from water workouts to fitness therapy. He was a frequent guest on both radio and print media on issues pertaining to senior fitness and the disabled.